YOUR BABY'S BOTTLE-FEEDING AVERSION

REASONS AND SOLUTIONS

ROWENA BENNETT

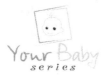

Your Baby
series

To my son, Hayden Bennett. Without your encouragement to publish an article on feeding aversions this book would never have happened. The response was phenomenal. After assisting hundreds by publishing just one article, I thought: let's help thousands through a book! Thank you Hayden for your encouragement and belief in me.

I also dedicate this book to parents who are desperately searching for a solution to their baby's bottle-feeding aversion.

YOUR BABY'S BOTTLE-FEEDING AVERSION

REASONS AND SOLUTIONS

ROWENA BENNETT

Registered nurse
Certified midwife
Certified mental health nurse
Certified child, adolescent and family health nurse
Graduate Diploma in Health Promotions
International Board Certified Lactation Consultant (IBCLC)

Published by Your Baby Series
PO Box 1260
Maroochydore Qld
AUSTRALIA
www.yourbabyseries.com

ISBN 978-0-6480984-0-9

Book formatting by www.finitepublishing.com

Other books by Rowena Bennett

Your Sleepless Baby

Also available in Spanish

Tu Bebé Desvelado

Available from leading online bookstores, Amazon and the author's websites.

www.yourbabyseries.com

www.babycareadvice.com

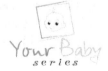

Contents

PART A: Identify the cause

What is a feeding aversion? • Signs • Causes • Being pressured • Bitter tasting formula or medications • Pain • Choking episodes • Medical trauma • Sensory processing disorder • Others

Major sucking problems • Barriers to effective sucking • How to choose suitable equipment • How to resolve airflow problems • How to position baby for feeding

How babies are pressured to feed • What happens when a baby is pressured • Why babies feed while sleeping • Why pressure is often overlooked as a cause of aversive feeding behavior

How to tell if pain is the cause • Physical problems that cause pain while feeding • Signs and symptoms • Treatments for conditions that cause feeding aversion • Misdiagnosis • The 'Medical Maze' and how to escape it

PART B: Correct misperceptions

PART C: Solutions

Important disclaimer

Your Baby's Bottle-feeding Aversion is designed to help parents and caregivers obtain general information about caring for, and promoting the health of babies and children. Information, opinions or judgments in this book are not intended as a substitute for medical advice. The content is provided for general use and may be unsuitable for babies or children suffering from certain conditions, diagnosed or otherwise.

Accordingly no person should rely on the contents of this book without first obtaining appropriate medical advice. This publication is sold entirely on the understanding that the author and/or consultants and/ or editors are not responsible for the results of any actions taken on the basis of information in this publication, nor for an error or omission from this publication, and further that the publisher is not engaged in rendering medical, pediatric, or professional or other advice or services. The publisher and author, consultants and editors expressly disclaim all liability to any person, whether a purchaser or reader of this publication or not, in respect to anything and of the consequences of anything done or omitted to be done by any such person in reliance whether wholly or partially upon the whole or any part of the contents of this publication. Without limiting the generality of the above, no author, consultant or editor shall have any responsibility for any act or omission of any other author, consultant or editor.

About the author

My husband Bruce and I live on the Sunshine Coast in Queensland, Australia. We have three adult children, Hayden, Jessica and Caitlin, and five adorable grandchildren, Elijah, Willow, Harlow, Isla and Bodhi. I naively thought life would get quieter as I got older, but the more grandchildren that arrive, the busier I become. I love spending time with family and friends, traveling, cycling, and riding my scooter, Lola.

I provide an online consultation service – **www.babycareadvice.com** – for parents living around the globe (provided they speak English). Consultations relate to infant crying, feeding and sleeping problems. I love chatting with parents about their babies, so it doesn't feel like work. I also enjoy writing about baby health issues and problems experienced by healthy babies which I publish on my website, **www.babycareadvice.com**. My first book, called *Your Sleepless Baby*, as the name suggests, is about baby sleep problems and solutions. This was published in 2012.

Professional qualifications

I have always enjoyed learning. During my nursing career, which has so far spanned over 40 years, I have gained professional qualifications as a registered nurse, midwife, mental health nurse, pediatric and child health nurse, I am an International Board Certified Lactation Consultant (IBCLC) and have a graduate diploma in Health Promotions. That's over 8½ years of tertiary education (university or college level).

Bottle-feeding aversion experience

Australia is one of only a handful of countries that train child health nurses to facilitate well-baby health checks and provide health information and parenting advice related to babies and children up to the age of 18 years. The Australian government also funds a number of child health early parenting education centers, where parents and their babies and young children are admitted to stay for five days. During this time they receive 24-hour, hands-on support from qualified child health nurses to assist them to resolve well-baby or child care problems, such as feeding and sleeping problems.

I was employed as a child health nurse in a child health early parenting education center for approximately 18 years. During that time, I learned about child development, how it relates to feeding and nutrition, and the causes and solutions to different types of infant feeding problems. I have had innumerable opportunities to bottle-feed babies, observe parents feeding their babies and witness how babies respond to different feeding techniques. I had previously trained as a mental health nurse and studied the many theories on learned behavior. Working closely with families at the parenting education center I could see how parents' actions influenced their child's behavior, and how certain infant feeding practices would reinforce or discourage desirable and undesirable behavior, including aversive feeding behavior.

From my experience at the parenting education center, I knew it was not essential to see a physically well baby to identify the reason for crying, feeding or sleeping problems. I just needed to know which questions to ask parents. And so, in 2002 I decided to start an online consultation service. I developed feeding plans to resolve behavioral feeding aversions. As a result of my successes, word spread in parenting forums, and I had a steady flow of feeding aversion cases as well as other baby care problems. After posting an article on feeding aversion on my website in 2013, the number of cases I assisted with, quadrupled. Feeding aversion is now the most common reason for consultations booked through my website. To date, I have been involved with over 1000 cases. Eighty percent relate to bottle-feeding aversion and the rest to breastfeeding and solids.

Why I wrote this book

Parents don't seek an online parenting consultation service as the first option when faced with an infant feeding problem. Most of my clients claimed to have consulted between three and seven, and some up to 15 health professionals from various fields before discovering my website.

Many of my clients express feelings or frustration and anger over their fruitless search for an effective solution. They explain how they shed tears time and time again as they witness how upset their precious baby becomes at feeding times as he or she frantically tries to avoid feeding despite obvious signs of hunger. Some pray daily for relief from the constant stress.

Many feel socially isolated because their baby won't feed except when sleeping. They lie in bed at the end of each day and wonder how they will make it through another day. But they do, because of the love they feel for their baby. They are tireless in their pursuit for answers.

Despite all they have suffered, my clients are among the lucky ones. Most are able to reverse their baby's feeding aversion and get back to the joy of watching their baby get excited by the sight of a bottle when hungry, and feed contentedly in their arms.

What saddens me is that countless families are not so lucky. The cause of their baby's bottle-feeding aversion is not identified or not managed effectively and so it continues, or as can often be the case, deteriorates further. The child may also become averse to eating solids, experience growth problems, and for a small percentage, require tube feeding.

I don't plan on providing consultations forever. And the number I can provide will become less as more grandchildren arrive, my husband retires and we travel more. So before I'm either too busy or too old to spend months writing what I have learned, I decided I had to write this book. I do so in the hope that I can help even more babies return to enjoyable feeding. It's so important to their whole family that they do.

If your family's life is burdened as a result of your baby's aversion to bottle-feeding, I truly hope that you find the answers you seek within these pages. I think you will.

Acknowledgments

So many parents shared their time, and often their tears, to tell the stories in this book. I feel humbled by their display of faith in allowing me to guide them out of the nightmare they endured for weeks or months as a result of their baby's feeding aversion. I feel privileged to have become a part of their story. I thank them all.

However, there would be no telling any of their stories if it was not for my son, Hayden Bennett. Hayden encouraged me to publish an article on feeding aversions on my website. Having done so, the number of feeding aversion cases I was involved with rose significantly. The confidence I gained from assisting hundreds of parents to successfully resolve their baby's feeding aversion has enabled me to write this book.

I would also like to thank my editor, Jessica Perini. Without her support and guidance, I am not sure if I would have completed this book. While I have extensive experience in verbally advising parents how to resolve their baby's bottle-feeding aversion, writing about it was a different matter. There were times I felt lost in the complexity of writing about this problem. Jessica has amazing insight. Even though she was not familiar with the topic, she was able to see the bigger picture and guide me.

Introduction

Sarah's story

We have tried everything to fix Jacob's feeding problem. We have seen a pediatrician, GI specialist, ENT specialist, speech and language pathologist, occupational therapist, tried three medications, four baby formulas and every different bottle and nipple we could find, but nothing has worked. Because Jacob looks healthy and his weight is okay, his doctor said, "Keep doing what you're doing." I went home and burst into tears. I am at breaking point. I don't know how much longer I can go on.

Jacob's feeding rules our lives. We can't leave the house because I don't want to miss the chance to feed him. He screams when I put him into a feeding position. Every feed is a battle that ends with both of us in tears. He's not sleeping well because I have to try to feed him in his sleep if he doesn't drink enough while awake. He often wakes up while I am trying to feed him. I feel like I am in a constant state of anxiety. Even when he's not feeding I am thinking about his last feed and whether or not he will eat next feed. I'm not sleeping because I wake up in the night and worry what the next day will be like. I worry about him getting dehydrated or sick if I can't get enough milk into him. I count every ounce, and how many more opportunities there will be to squeeze in another feed before bedtime. I worry how the stress is affecting our relationship. I fear he will learn to hate me. I don't know how I am going to go back to work because he won't eat for anyone else but me. If I don't work, we won't be able to pay the mortgage. My mood swings depending on whether Jacob has had a good feeding day or not. I have been diagnosed with depression, but I honestly think if Jacob was feeding better, I would feel fine.

If Sarah's story sounds similar to your own, it could be that your baby has developed an aversion to bottle-feeding. If that's the case then this book is for you.

Bottle-feeding aversion

An aversion refers to a **psychological or emotional response** where a person tries to avoid an object or situation. A feeding phobia is another term sometimes used to explain baby's distress and avoidance of feeding.

Babies become apprehensive or fearful if the experience of feeding is often unpleasant, stressful or painful.

Babies as young as two months of age will try to avoid a situation they fear. As babies mature, their memory develops, they become increasingly more aware of their environment and the circumstances surrounding feeding, and they become more skilled at avoiding feeding should they chose to do so. Babies who have developed an aversion to feeding appear as if they would rather starve than eat. Once averse to feeding they don't willingly eat enough, except when sleeping, and sleep-feeding eventually becomes ineffective.

An infant feeding aversion is one of the most stressful, confusing, frustrating and complex problems a parent could face. As a result, parents often lose confidence in their parenting ability and second-guess every decision they make regarding their baby's feeding.

It's estimated that between 25 to 45 percent of otherwise normal-developing babies have feeding problems.[1] This includes all forms of feeding aversion – bottle-feeding, breastfeeding and solids – plus other feeding problems experienced by babies **who are capable of feeding**.

The percentage of babies troubled by a bottle-feeding aversion has not been established. One reason could be because **it's a poorly recognized problem**. Many people mistakenly assume that babies are too young to develop a negative psychological response to experiences that occur while feeding. Consequently, this limits their search for reasons and solutions to babies' distressed feeding behavior to physical or medical causes.

Failure to accurately identify the cause results in ineffective treatment plans. This means a baby's feeding aversion can continue for months or years. If the cause of baby's bottle-feeding aversion is not identified and corrected, the same cause can lead to an aversion to eating solids foods as well.

The good news is that **a feeding aversion is a reversible problem.** If an effective solution has not yet been presented to you – hence why you're reading this book – the reason for your baby's oppositional feeding behavior may not as yet been correctly identified, or multiple causes may be involved, or the strategies recommended so far are unhelpful or counterproductive.

As you have not received answers from the various health professionals you have already consulted, it's up to you to discover the cause and solution. This book can show you how.

WARNING: If your baby is averse to bottle-feeding, the way you manage his feeds may have contributed to this problem. This realization could be very upsetting. Don't despair, help is here.

What's in this book?

While **your goal** in reading this book is to find a way for your baby to enjoy bottle-feeding and eat enough for healthy growth – **my goal** in writing this book is that you will achieve this and so much more. I hope that you will gain a greater understanding of your baby's needs and a deeper connection with him as a result of what you learn from reading this book.

Knowledge is the key to resolving your baby's feeding aversion. The problem is: we don't know what we don't know. This book is designed to provide the information that you may not be aware you're missing. The chapters are divided into three parts:

- Part A: Identify the cause
- Part B: Correct misperceptions
- Part C: Solutions

I encourage you to read all chapters in order, as they're structured to assist you to understand the situation, prepare you for the solutions that follow, and improve your chances of successfully resolving your baby's feeding aversion.

Here's a sample of what each part contains.

Part A: Identify the cause

The solution to an infant feeding aversion depends on **accurate** identification of the cause. The many possible causes can be divided into two broad groups:

1. **Behavioral** reasons (also called psychological) include unpleasant and stressful feeding experiences **without** pain.

2. **Physical** reasons include physical problems or medical conditions that make feeding uncomfortable or painful.

Behavioral reasons

The most common of all **behavioral reasons** for babies and children to become averse to feeding or eating is because they're pressured or forced to eat against their will. This makes the experience of bottle-feeding distressing for babies (and parents). When repeated, baby learns to anticipate the pressure and becomes tense and upset as soon as he recognizes the circumstances where he has been pressured in the past. This could be when a bib is placed around his neck, when he's placed into a feeding position or after being burped.

No parent enjoys pressuring or forcing their baby to feed. But some do so out of loving concern because they fear something bad will happen to baby if they don't make sure he eats an expected amount.

Diagram: Fear-pressure-fear-avoidance cycle

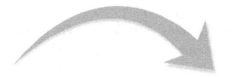

Parents fear something bad will happen to baby if he doesn't eat as much as expected and pressure him to eat.

Baby fears feeding because he has been repeatedly pressured to feed and refuses to eat or eats very little.

The more baby is pressured, the more he tries to avoid feeding. The more he tries to avoid feeding, the more anxious parents become and the more pressure they apply to make him feed, the longer feeding takes, and the more stressful the situation becomes for everyone involved. The more often a baby is pressured or forced to feed, the greater the chance he will become averse to feeding.

While being pressured to feed is the most common cause, babies can become fearful of feeding for other reasons, such as repeated choking episodes, the memory of painful or stressful medical procedures involving baby's mouth or face (even though feeding is not causing pain he fears it will), and sensory processing problems.

Physical reasons

There are a number of physical problems which **while untreated** can cause pain or discomfort while feeding and as a result cause a baby to become averse to feeding. These include:

- acid reflux
- milk protein allergy or intolerance or
- gastro-paresis (delayed gastric emptying time).

Only a **tiny** percentage of babies suffer from these conditions, but a **large** percentage of babies who become averse to feeding are diagnosed with these conditions and others during brief medical consultations. Overdiagnosis of these problems in respect to babies occurs because people in general, including most doctors, are unaware of **behavioral** reasons and solutions for infant feeding and sleeping problems.

If your search for answers to your baby's feeding aversion has provided no effective solution, it's time to consider ALL possible causes.

Chapters 1 to 4 provide information on how to recognize or rule out various causes of bottle-feeding aversion, and pinpoint the reason or reasons your baby no longer enjoys feeding.

Part B: Correct misperceptions

Everyone you meet will have an opinion on the cause and solution to your baby's feeding problems. You may have received advice from multiple sources already.

There are four areas in particular where health professionals make mistakes and as a consequence parents are poorly advised. These mistakes can cause or perpetuate infant feeding aversion.

- **Mistake 1:** Parents are taught to control rather than support their baby's feeding.
- **Mistake 2:** Baby's milk needs are overestimated.
- **Mistake 3:** Normal variations of growth are mistaken as poor growth.
- **Mistake 4:** It's assumed that poor growth – whether real or perceived – is because baby is not eating enough.

Babies who don't follow a typical growth pattern, such as preterm babies, intra-uterine growth restricted (IUGR) babies, genetically short statured babies, babies born very large, babies who overfeed or underfeed in the early weeks, genetically lean babies, and others have an increased risk of developing a feeding aversion for the reasons above.

As you read through the pages of this book you will notice numerous examples of health professionals getting it wrong, of mistaken assumptions, misdiagnoses, and poor advice given to parents. I acknowledge that I am only consulted about feeding aversion cases that other health professionals have been unable to solve. I don't get to see the countless families who receive a correct diagnosis and good advice from their healthcare professionals.

If you're reading this book, you may have misperceptions about your responsibilities when feeding your baby or you may have been misinformed about your baby's milk needs or expected growth. If mistaken beliefs are not identified and corrected, these may prevent you from making the changes in infant feeding practices required to resolve your baby's aversion.

Chapters 5 to 9 may help you define your responsibilities when feeding your baby, clarify your expectations regarding his milk needs and growth, and better understand why this unfortunate situation has developed.

Part C: Solutions

I know you would love a cure that will suddenly switch your baby from avoidance to willing feeding. But that doesn't happen in the case of a feeding aversion. An aversion to feeding can be resolved, but there is no quick fix.

Irrespective of the original cause of a baby's feeding refusal, it's likely he has been pressured to feed in subtle or obvious ways. The fear-pressure-fear-avoidance cycle damages the parent–child feeding relationship, but not irrevocably.

There's usually a loss of trust on both sides. The parent doesn't trust baby to eat enough for healthy growth and baby doesn't trust a parent or both parents to respond in harmony with his wishes. Even after parents stop pressuring their baby to eat, it takes time to restore baby's trust. And trust must be restored before baby will willingly eat enough for healthy growth.

Chapters 9 to 15 describe my **Five Steps to Success** which include feeding rules and recommendations to support your baby to get over his fear of feeding and learn that feeding is enjoyable. Also included is what to expect as your baby recovers, how to support baby's sleep throughout the process, how to tell if things are on track, what to do if they're not, and what life might be like when baby is over his aversion.

Note: All case studies in this book are real, but names have been changed. The words 'he' and 'she' are used in alternate chapters. The term 'parents' also applies to caregivers who feed babies.

As a health professional, I know the importance of evidence-based practice. However, so little is written about bottle-feeding aversion, as you have no doubt also discovered. So references will be scant. **My feeding rules** have a strong evidence base to support their effectiveness as a way to encourage healthy relationships with food and eating. (You will find references in the back of this book.)

My feeding recommendations are based on many years of experience, learning what works and what doesn't, and tweaking feeding plans until achieving a high success rate.

Who may find this book helpful?

- **Babies** will benefit the most from their parents reading this book and adapting their infant feeding practices in ways that promote their baby's enjoyment of feeding.
- **Parents** of babies who are averse to bottle-feeding will gain a greater understanding of how they influence their baby's feeding behavior for better or worse, and how to end the nightmare of an infant feeding aversion.
- **Health professionals** who are asked to advise on the reason for bottle-refusal and/or provide infant feeding advice to parents, such as general practitioners, pediatricians, pediatric medical specialists, midwives, pediatric nurses, community health nurses, speech and language pathologists, occupational therapists, and pediatric dietitians, may gain a greater understanding of behavioral reasons and solutions for infant feeding aversion.

- **Child-care workers** who come into contact with babies who are averse to bottle-feeding may become more aware of infant feeding aversion and as a result help the babies they care for by informing parents of the possibility of this problem.

What's not covered in this book?

This book is specific to bottle-feeding aversion. While many of the guiding principles apply to other forms of feeding, such as breastfeeding, solids or tube-feeding, other feeding methods are not covered.

The feeding recommendations in this book apply to **babies who have the physical capacity to feed well** from a bottle, but who are presently refusing because they're averse to feeding. Feeding recommendations for special needs babies, those who have neurological problems or congenital disabilities that make it difficult for them to feed, are not covered. However, special needs babies are at increased risk for both behavioral and physical reasons for feeding aversion. So, if your special needs baby has become averse to feeding, the information in this book may still apply.

PART A:
Identify the cause

1

Bottle-feeding aversion causes

> Feeding Amelia (aged four months) has become a nightmare. She acts like I am trying to poison her. I just have to lay her in my arms and she goes ballistic. I don't understand why. She used to gobble her feeds down until about two months ago. Things have gotten MUCH worse in the past month. Now I have to fight with her to get her to drink. I hate doing it but I am so worried she's going to end up with a feeding tube. I don't know what to do. I'm desperate. Do you think you can help? – Corinne

Based on Corinne's description, I suspect Amelia has developed a feeding aversion. A baby can become averse to bottle-feeding for numerous reasons. Before Corinne can remedy the situation, she needs to figure out what's troubling Amelia. To achieve this it's necessary for her to learn what a feeding aversion is, and the various reasons babies become averse to feeding.

Let's look at the first vital step involved in resolving an infant feeding aversion: **exploring all possible causes.** By doing so, you can begin the process of eliminating these one by one until you have pinpointed the triggers causing your baby's aversive feeding behavior.

What is a feeding aversion?

An aversion involves an avoidance of a thing or situation because it's associated with an unpleasant, stressful or painful stimulus. An infant bottle-feeding aversion is where a baby – **who can physically feed from a bottle** – partially or completely refuses to feed. Babies can develop an aversion to breastfeeding, bottle-feeding and/or eating solid foods. Some babies become averse to just one method of feeding, others two or all three.

In the case of a feeding aversion, baby's oppositional behavior at feeding times becomes a conditioned response. Initially, baby becomes upset in direct response to the **stimulus** – the thing or circumstance causing the feeding experience to be unpleasant, stressful or painful. For example, stress associated with being pressured to feed against her will, or pain while swallowing caused by acid reflux or milk allergy. After repeated exposure she learns to link the act of feeding or eating with the stimulus (eg, being pressured or pain) and becomes tense or upset in anticipation.

Signs that baby may be averse to feeding

If your baby has developed an aversion to bottle-feeding she might exhibit some of the following behaviors:

- Appears hungry but refuses to eat.
- Reluctantly eats only when ravenous and then takes only a small amount.
- Becomes tense, cries or screams when a bib is placed around her neck, when placed into a feeding position, or when shown the bottle, or after stopping to burp.
- Clamps her mouth shut and turns her head away from the bottle.
- Takes a few sips or a small portion of milk and pulls away or arches back and starts to cry.
- Consumes less milk than expected.
- Avoids eye contact while feeding.
- Rejects feeding while held in arms.

- Moves the nipple around her mouth with her tongue and refuses to drink.
- Fights being fed with every ounce of her strength until she's too tired to fight any longer.
- Feeds only while in a drowsy state or asleep.
- Accepts milk from a dropper, syringe, spoon or sippy cup or enthusiastically eats solid foods after refusing to drink from the bottle.
- Displays poor growth or has been diagnosed as 'failure to thrive'.

The type and intensity of behavior varies between babies. This relates to a baby's age, temperament and the lengths to which parents go to make their baby feed.

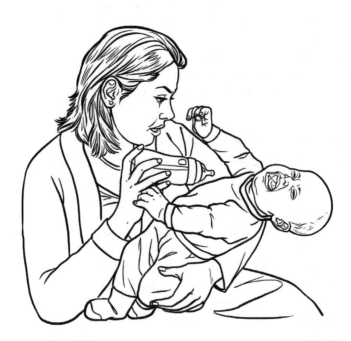

> **Conflicted feeding behavior**
>
> Babies who have a feeding aversion will often display conflicted feeding behavior. 'Conflicted' because it appears like baby doesn't know what she wants to do. She's tense but accepts the bottle, takes a few sucks, turns away or back arches in an agitated state. Within seconds she turns back and indicates she wants the bottle again. She takes a few more sucks, pulls away upset, but quickly returns and so on. She could repeat this behavior throughout the feed or until she becomes drowsy, at which time she might feed well.

Why aversive feeding behavior persists

Behavior that is reinforced will continue. If a baby's avoidant feeding behavior is no longer reinforced it will gradually fade in intensity and disappear within a matter of days or weeks.

An essential key to resolving your baby's feeding aversion is to **accurately identify and eliminate the stimulus.** Failure to do so means her behavior could continue to be reinforced for weeks, months or years.

Accurate identification of the stimulus requires a **thorough** assessment. The fact that baby fusses **prior to** the stimulus makes it challenging to figure out what she is reacting to. Only baby knows what's upsetting her and she can't tell anyone. Others can only make **assumptions** or **guesses** about the cause. How much information they gather about the circumstances surrounding baby's avoidant feeding behavior, in particular how the parents act **before and after** baby objects to feeding and how she behaves at times unrelated to feeding, will determine whether their guess is a stab in the dark or on target.

A book is not the first place any parent would look for answers to an infant feeding problem. You have probably consulted with one or multiple health professionals in your search for a solution. Hence, your baby may have already received one or more diagnoses to explain why she tries to avoid feeding. If her aversive feeding behavior has continued weeks after commencing treatment or feeding therapy, this indicates her behavior continues to be reinforced.

One or both of the following reasons could be responsible:

- a mistaken assumption about the cause or
- ineffective treatment or removal of the cause.

The first step is to accurately pinpoint the cause.

Causes

Aversive behavior can be triggered by a single highly traumatic event. But more often babies become averse to feeding because they are repeatedly exposed to feeding experiences that are unpleasant, stressful or painful.

Babies can become upset, frightened or stressed at feeding times for different reasons including:

- being pressured to feed
- bitter tasting formula, breast milk or medicine
- pain
- choking episodes
- medical trauma
- sensory processing disorder.

We'll examine these causes below.

Being pressured to feed

We have all done it at some point. We think we're encouraging baby to take a little more because we don't think she's had enough. But in reality we're using gentle or not so gentle forms of pressure to make her feed after she indicates she wants to stop. Even subtle forms of pressure – commonly considered as 'encouragement' or 'helping' baby to feed – can be enough to cause and/or reinforce a baby's feeding aversion.

Pressuring a baby or child to feed or eat is THE most common cause of feeding aversion. More often than not I find that pressure is the **original and only cause** of a baby's avoidant feeding behavior. However, pressure can also be a **secondary** cause that reinforces a baby's aversion long after the original cause has resolved. For example, a baby might originally object to feeding due to pain associated with acid reflux. In response to her feeding refusal, her parent then pressures her. Pain is effectively relieved by medications, but her objection to feeding continues because she has now learned to link feeding with the stress of being pressured to feed.

Being pressured to feed was the original and only cause of Madison's aversive feeding behavior. Her mother, Lauren, described the situation below.

Lauren's comments

From week six Maddy started to reject the bottle despite showing hunger cues. The situation has gotten worse since then. She was taking 28 ounces (oz) until week nine and ever since it is 21 oz on average. When she first started to reject we thought it might be linked to silent reflux. The GP prescribed Gaviscon (an antacid) then Ranitidine (an acid suppressing medication) to see if these would fix the problem. She was on Ranitidine for a month but there was no improvement.

Last month we were referred to a pediatrician who suggested we try giving her Elecare (a hypoallergenic formula) and Omeprazole (an even more potent acid suppressing medication). She hated the taste of Elecare and would even reject it in sleep feeds, which up until then had been the only time we managed to get her to drink a decent amount. We only managed to completely switch her formula last week. But since being on Elecare and Omeprazole there has been no improvement either, and the feeding process remains very difficult. We also took her to a chiropractor (four times in total over a period of six weeks). There was a short-term improvement after the first couple of appointments in terms of her seeming slightly calmer. However, this didn't last and the subsequent appointments have made no improvement.

Now (aged four months) Maddy reacts aggressively right from the moment we pick her up to hold her to feed. She often reacts like this even when it is not feeding time. Typically, she straightens her legs, arches her back, turns her head from side to side while screaming and rejects the bottle. If we stop trying to feed her and change her position she stops screaming but continues to cry because she's hungry. The only way to get her to feed is to rock her to sleep first, and then feed. However, getting her to sleep when she is distressed because of hunger is a very lengthy and difficult process. It can take up to 90 minutes to settle her to sleep and finally get her to drink her milk. At night it's easier.

> Nights have been good in comparison to the daytime. At night she feeds just fine. Whilst we feel this is because she is half asleep, it has at least enabled us to get some rest, as her day feeds have become incredibly difficult to manage.
>
> I am desperate for Maddy to feed like a normal baby with stress-free feeding while awake. I would like to regain some normality to our lives without the long drawn out feeding process and be able to do other things. I would like to feel confident again when feeding my baby and to go out more without worrying about feeding her while being out of the house.

Maddy's feeding issues were behavioral. She reacted in this way because Lauren overlooked her cues that indicated she was finished eating while trying to make her drink the amount recommended on the formula can. As a result of being repeatedly pressured to eat, Maddy became averse to feeding and was then not eating enough. Maddy did not have acid reflux or milk protein intolerance. Once her feeding aversion was resolved using the methods described in this book, medications were ceased and she was switched back to a regular baby formula with no ill effects.

'Pressure' is described in greater detail in Chapter 3.

Bitter tasting medicine, formula or breast milk

Nasty tasting medicine given directly before feeds or given using nipple-shaped devices, or added into a baby's bottle could cause rejection of bottle-feeds, more so if baby is forced to take the medicine.

A sudden switch from the sweet taste of breast milk to infant formula or to the bitter taste of hypoallergenic formula can cause a baby to reject feeds. While the unpleasant taste of a new formula might cause baby's initial rejection of bottle-feeds, usually a baby will come around to accepting it provided she's not pressured to feed. However, opposition to the change in taste could lead to baby being pressured to eat. Feeding refusal over the long term is more likely to be caused by pressure rather than the taste of the formula.

Breast milk typically has a sweet taste. However, a small percentage of breastfeeding mothers produce excess amounts of lipase in their breast milk. (Lipase is an enzyme that breaks down fats in breast milk to help baby digest it.) The breakdown of fats begins soon after the milk is pumped. When lipase is in excess this process occurs more rapidly causing the milk to smell or taste rancid, soapy or metallic. The milk is safe for baby to drink but some babies don't like the taste. For some women it only takes a few hours before the milk fats break down enough to alter the taste, for others it could be 24 hours. Fortunately, lipase can be inactivated at high temperatures, and milk can be safely stored in a refrigerator or freezer. Milk must be scalded before freezing, as lipase is still active even at low temperatures. If pumped breast milk doesn't smell distinctly sour or rancid, then the taste is probably not the reason for your baby to fuss or reject bottle-feeds.

Pain

A number of physical problems and medical conditions can make it painful for babies to feed and cause fear of feeding. The following conditions are commonly blamed, but seldom responsible, for babies' aversive feeding behavior:

- acid reflux
- milk allergy or intolerance
- gastro-paresis (delayed gastric emptying)
- constipation
- mouth ulcers
- oral thrush and
- teething.

Chapter 4 explains how you can tell if these conditions are the cause of your baby's avoidant feeding behavior.

Choking episodes

A baby could reject feeds owing to fright as a result of a single traumatic choking episode or repeated choking episodes. If choking were the cause then baby would exhibit aversive behavior directly following the event. But remember, behavior must be reinforced. So if baby experiences repeated feeds where there is no choking, her negative feelings about feeding will wane and disappear.

If on the other hand, she periodically experiences further stressful episodes of choking, this could reinforce her determination to avoid feeding and the stress associated with choking. Chapter 2 explains how to prevent choking episodes.

Medical trauma

Unpleasant or invasive medical interventions such as nasal or oral suctioning, feeding tube insertion, or intubation can cause a baby to become frightened when anything comes near her face. From these experiences she may learn that things that touch her face or mouth cause pain and so she becomes upset when the nipple of a bottle is placed into her mouth.

If a baby's avoidant feeding behavior is due to these reasons, she will display such behavior **directly** following the event. Her behavior may be reinforced while these procedures are repeated. Rest assured, once these events pass any reluctance to feed caused by these procedures will also pass within days or weeks.

Sensory processing disorder

Babies can develop an **oral aversion** due to a **sensory processing disorder**. Babies who have such a disorder perceive sensations differently to others and become upset by situations and things that don't trouble most other babies. They may find a particular smell, taste or feel of certain foods or feel of the nipple of the bottle and other objects in their mouth objectionable. Or they may be less aware or hypersensitive to the sensation of hunger.

Babies **formally diagnosed** with sensory processing disorder – based on specific types of behavior that point to this problem – may benefit from treatment provided by an occupational therapist. When a baby is believed to be troubled by the sensation of having the nipple of a bottle in her mouth, treatment may include putting an Oro-Navigator or Probe Tip, both of which look a little like a rubbery toothbrush with ridges or bumps rather than bristles, into baby's mouth to desensitize her to the feel of things in her mouth.

Oral aversion versus feeding aversion

Oral aversion is not the same as a feeding aversion. In the case of an oral aversion, a baby typically objects to anything in her mouth including the nipple of a feeding bottle. Whereas in the case of a bottle-feeding aversion, baby is happy to have things in her mouth just so long as it's not the nipple of a bottle (or breast or solids in the case of these types of feeding aversions) which she has learned to associate with stress or pain.

Misdiagnosis of a sensory processing disorder or oral aversion as the cause of a baby's aversive feeding behavior that develops as a result of being repeatedly pressured to feed, is common. In the case of bottle-feeding aversion, rarely is the cause of feeding refusal related to the feel of the nipple in baby's mouth or a sensory processing disorder. If your baby has a history of feeding well, plus she's also willing to have other things in her mouth, such as a pacifier, fingers, toys, it's unlikely that her refusal to drink from a bottle is due to oral aversion.

A sensory processing disorder is **one of the least common causes** of feeding aversion. It's not possible to accurately diagnose a sensory processing disorder based on a baby's aversive feeding behavior **before** behavioral feeding aversion therapy (such as the process described in this book) has been implemented and **given sufficient time** to reverse any negative feelings baby has about feeding.

If the cause of your baby's aversive feeding behavior is due to pressure or another reason, desensitization treatment for oral aversion is unhelpful and potentially counterproductive. Putting things into your baby's mouth without her permission could reinforce her aversive feeding behavior.

Other causes

Babies can find feeding to be unpleasant, frightening or stressful for other reasons. For example, feeding in a highly stimulating environment, loud noise, lots of people talking, a toddler periodically touching, bumping or poking baby while she's feeding, and more. Any feeding situation that results in a baby becoming upset, frightened or stressed, when repeated can trigger apprehension around feeding or an aversion to feeding.

Identify the cause

An **effective** solution to an infant feeding aversion means any feeding strategy or treatment MUST remove the stimulus reinforcing baby's feeding refusal. The most likely reason you have not yet found a solution is because the trigger for your baby's continued resistance to feeding has not yet been identified or not effectively removed.

While any of the causes mentioned could be the reason a baby first objects to feeding, **in 100 percent of bottle-feeding aversion cases I have been involved with, the baby was pressured to feed.** However, not all parents were aware that the infant feeding strategies they employed involved pressure. In the majority of cases, pressure was the original cause. In some cases, pressure reinforced baby's aversive feeding behavior long after the original cause had passed or had been effectively treated.

Before identifying if pressure is reinforcing your baby's oppositional feeding behavior it's important to rule out sucking problems. Chapter 2 explains what to look for.

2

Rule out sucking problems

> When Hugo first started to get upset during feeds, I thought he was having trouble sucking. We tried every bottle and nipple we could find, but it didn't seem to make much difference. I took him to a speech therapist who said he didn't appear to have trouble sucking. I am at a loss to know what his problem is. – Erica

With the help of a speech and language pathologist (SLP) Erica has determined that Hugo doesn't have issues that prevent him from sucking from a bottle. This is good because it means Erica no longer needs to worry about the possibility that Hugo **can't** feed effectively. She can now focus on figuring out why he **doesn't want to** feed.

Some babies can have major sucking problems related to their sucking ability, or more specifically inability to suck properly. They can also experience frustration due to equipment problems or the way they're fed. Before confirming if your baby has an aversion, you need to rule out sucking problems. But you don't necessarily need to see a speech therapist to achieve this. Once you know what signs to look for, a sucking problem will be apparent.

If your baby has a history of feeding well prior to objecting to feeding, or if he currently feeds well in a sleepy state, there's probably nothing wrong with the feeding equipment or his ability to suck. However, if you have concerns or would like to feel confident you've covered all bases then read on.

Major sucking problems

A number of physical problems can prevent a baby from feeding well:

- **Structural problems,** meaning baby has a physical abnormality affecting his face or mouth, such as cleft palate, small jaw or tongue-tie.
- **Functional problems** preventing baby from sucking properly. Problems affecting baby's brain or nervous system, for example cerebral palsy, brain hemorrhage, nerve damage or compression due to a traumatic birth, can result in an uncoordinated suck-swallow-breathe pattern, weak suck, or an absence of baby's sucking reflex.

If your baby has or had an abnormality or impairment that affects his ability to coordinate sucking, swallowing and breathing, this would have been identified soon after birth. In this case, an SLP is probably already involved in his care.

If your baby has sucking problems, the solution may be a matter of:

- choosing suitable feeding equipment to make feeding easier or
- thickening his feeds to prevent choking or
- switching to high-energy feeds to reduce the effort required to gain the calories he needs for healthy growth or
- feeding therapy to improve his sucking coordination.

Your baby's doctor or SLP will advise on the most appropriate course of action.

If you have concerns or doubts about your baby's ability to suck effectively, discuss this with his doctor, who can refer him to a speech and language pathologist for assessment, if necessary.

Barriers to effective sucking

A baby could be physically capable of feeding well and yet be prevented from doing so due to unsuitable or faulty feeding equipment, poor positioning or airflow problems. To overcome these potential barriers you may need to:

- choose suitable feeding equipment
- ensure continuous airflow within the bottle while baby feeds and
- provide appropriate positional support.

Choose suitable equipment

Even though a baby could be physically capable of feeding well, faulty or unsuitable equipment could make it difficult or impossible for him to feed effectively. But how do you know? By watching for unusual behavior like clicking, gagging, coughing or spluttering, or falling asleep before completing the feed. Such behavior might indicate an equipment problem.

Nipple size and shape

A baby could repeatedly **gag** if the shaft of the nipple (the part that sits in baby's mouth) is too long. He might make repeated **clicking sounds** due to loss of suction if the shaft is too short. But these are not the only causes of gagging and clicking. Gagging with or without vomiting is also common when a baby is forced to feed and it can become a conditioned response as a result of being repeatedly pressured. Clicking can also be related to a high or unusually shaped palate.

There are many feeding nipples to choose from. Most nipples fit within three broad categories:

- **Narrow-neck.** These have a bell shape and fit on a narrow bottle. I generally recommend these as the shape allows for a natural gape of baby's mouth and the shaft is usually a good length to enable baby to comfortably maintain suction.
- **Broad-based.** These have a domed appearance and fit on wide-necked bottles. I don't recommend these because I find the length of the shaft is too short for **some** babies. However, if your baby appears to suck well with a broad-based nipple, there's no need to switch.
- **Orthodontic.** These were designed to fill baby's mouth while feeding. Some babies prefer the shape of these nipples.

TIP: Don't believe claims made by manufacturers that a particular feeding nipple is just like a mother's nipple. No man-made latex or silicone nipple can replicate the shape and flexibility of a breastfeeding mother's nipple.

Flow rate

If the rate at which milk flows through the hole at the end of the nipple is too fast it could cause baby to **cough or splutter** and frighten him. Even when a baby appears to cope with the flow rate, a nipple that is too fast could cause him to **swallow a lot of air**. Feeding too quickly (also called speed-feeding) is a major cause of overfeeding, as described in Chapter 5. Alternatively, if the flow rate is too slow it could **frustrate** him or he could **tire and stop** before he's had enough.

Manufacturers usually provide a guide to flow rates by labeling nipples as:

- **Preterm:** for babies before they reach their expected date of birth
- **Slow, Newborn or Stage 1:** for babies from birth to three months
- **Medium or Stage 2:** for babies three to six months
- **Fast or Stage 3:** for babies over six months.

Consider these as a **guide only**. Even if you choose a nipple recommended for your baby's age, this doesn't mean it will be right for him. Babies of the same age vary in size, strength and sucking ability. Some babies suck with more or less vigor than others. The time it takes for your baby to complete a feed, when feeding well, can give you an idea of whether the flow rate is suitable or not.

How long is ideal feeding time?

As a general rule, the younger the baby, the slower the feed needs to be. I recommend you aim for the following timeframes while bottle-feeding your baby:

- **Birth to three months:** 20 to 40 minutes
- **Three months to six months:** 10 to 20 minutes
- **Over six months:** five to 15 minutes.

Please note: These timeframes don't imply that this is how long you should persist in feeding your baby. Rather they're an approximation of how long it might take your baby to comfortably **complete a reasonably sized feed** for his age and size, when feeding well.

- **If baby feeds too fast:** Choose a slower nipple.
- **If baby feeds too slowly:** First check that the issue is not poor positioning or an airflow problem. Once you have ruled out these problems, try a faster nipple.

If your baby only takes a small amount at each feed the timeframes may be shorter.

Resolve airflow problems

Non-vented bottles or nipples

To avoid leakage of milk, parents usually secure the nipple to the bottle by firmly screwing down the nipple ring. This can affect the rate of flow of milk from **non-vented bottles or nipples,** and can cause fussy feeding behavior or insufficient milk intake. It can also cause the nipple to collapse in baby's mouth.

The solution is simple. Loosen the nipple ring enough to allow air to enter the bottle between the rim of the bottle and base of the nipple. This will maintain a neutral pressure and a constant rate of flow throughout the entire feed. This tiny detail can make feeding easier, less frustrating and more enjoyable for a baby.

It can take practice to find the sweet spot between too tight and too loose. You can get a little leakage when you tip the bottle even when you have it right. You will know you have it right when you see a steady flow of bubbles into the bottle while your baby is feeding. There should be no rush of bubbles into the bottle when he releases suction by letting go of the nipple.

Alternatively, use a vented bottle or nipple.

Vented bottles and nipples

Vented bottles and nipples have inbuilt mechanisms that help maintain neutral air pressure within the bottle, but these are not fail proof. If your baby is using vented feeding equipment, bottles or nipples, check it's working properly. There should be no rush of bubbles into the bottle as your baby lets go. If there is, the venting system is not working properly. Make sure parts are attached correctly and not screwed on too tightly.

Ensure good feeding position

Poor positioning while feeding can impede a baby's ability to suck effectively. Examples of poor positioning include:

- baby's head is twisted to the side
- his head is pushed forward and his chin is pressed against his chest
- his head is tilted too far back
- he's flat on his back.

A newborn baby needs more support to position his body in a comfortable way while feeding compared to when he's three months of age or older. As a baby matures, he becomes stronger and more capable of supporting his head and moving his body into a comfortable position.

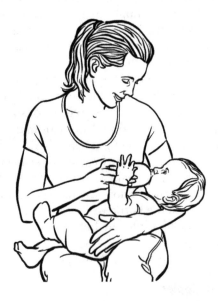

Position baby in a semi-reclined position at roughly a 45-degree angle on your lap so that he can look at you as he feeds. His head is in line with his body and resting in the crook of your arm. Hold him securely to prevent falling, but not restrictively. Don't restrain his head or limb movements.

This means no swaddling at feeding times, no tucking one of his arms behind your back or holding his wrist to prevent him from moving his arm, and no restricting his head movement.

Babies who have developed a feeding aversion might reject feeding in arms and may avoid eye contact while feeding. This situation will likely improve as you resolve your baby's feeding aversion using my feeding recommendations described in Chapters 9 to 11.

Now that you have ruled out sucking problems, the next step is to determine if pressure is the cause of your baby's oppositional feeding behavior.

3
Is pressure the cause?

> Arianna could be crying because of hunger, but
> as soon as I put her on her back in my arms to
> offer her the bottle she screams, tries to push it
> away, and buries her face into my chest. I have to
> walk her around and distract her with her pacifier
> to calm her down. I then switch the pacifier for
> the bottle. She might start screaming again and
> I have to calm her down again. I might have to do
> this three or four times. Eventually she will take
> an ounce or two (30-60 ml) and I dream feed the
> rest of her bottle when she naps. – Naomi

When asked, Naomi acknowledged she had been pressuring Arianna
to feed. As I explained to her why pressuring a baby to feed can
cause her to become averse to feeding, tears rolled down her cheeks.
The realization that – despite good intentions – she had unknowingly
caused Arianna to become fearful of feeding caused her anguish. I felt
dreadful that my words triggered her tears, but it was essential that
she recognize the cause of her baby's behavior, so she could change her
feeding practices and resolve Arianna's feeding aversion.

Being pressured to eat is – without exception – the most common
reason for healthy babies and children to become averse to feeding. If
pressure is the cause of your baby's aversive feeding behavior, then as
painful as this might be for you to accept, you need to acknowledge
this so that you can remedy the situation.

What constitutes 'pressure'?

'Pressure' includes anything that a parent might do to make a baby eat when she doesn't want to. If you disregard or overlook your baby's behavioral cues that indicate she wants to stop feeding and you keep trying to get her to drink more, this will undoubtedly involve some form of pressure.

Satiety cues: signs that baby has had enough

- Stops sucking.
- Pushing the nipple out of her mouth with her tongue.
- Turning her head away or arching back.
- Pushing the bottle away with her hand.
- Clamping her mouth shut.

Pressuring a baby or child to feed or eat can cause her to develop a behavioral feeding aversion. By 'behavioral' I am not implying that a baby acts in a deliberate, naughty or manipulative manner, rather that her aversive feeding behavior **occurs as a consequence** of the circumstances – in this instance due to being repeatedly pressured to feed – rather than a physical cause.

In regards to feeding a baby, there are varying degrees of pressure ranging from coercion, considered by many as 'encouragement', to force-feeding. Understanding how force-feeding would turn a baby off feeding makes its easier to appreciate why coercion could have a similar effect.

Force-feeding

Force-feeding involves a bigger, stronger, person exerting their will over a smaller, weaker person. Cassie's case shows how a chain of events can lead to a parent force-feeding their baby.

Baby Cassie

Cassie was born at 30 weeks gestation (10 weeks early). She progressed well without any serious complications. She was discharged from the maternity hospital, fully bottle-feeding, one week before her expected due date. Before discharge, her mother, Amanda, was shown how to encourage her to continue feeding by applying pressure under her chin. (This transfers pressure from the nipple to the roof of baby's mouth and triggers a newborn's sucking reflex.) By doing so, Amanda found she could get Cassie to take the recommended amount of milk. Cassie fed well for the first four weeks following discharge. She would occasionally projectile vomit what appeared like a large amount of milk, but this was not considered to be a problem as she was gaining weight well and she was relatively content except for minor fussiness during feeds.

Around six weeks adjusted age (the age she would have been had she been born around the time of her expected date of birth), Cassie became increasingly more difficult to feed. She would stop feeding and try to push the nipple out of her mouth. The more Cassie resisted, the longer Amanda found she needed to persist to ensure she drank the recommended amount. The number of times Cassie threw up milk increased. Cassie's doctor suspected acid reflux, and prescribed Omeprazole. This didn't improve the situation.

As the weeks progressed the battles over feeding became even more intense. By three months adjusted age vomiting had increased and she was diagnosed with delayed gastric emptying and given Domperidone (a medication that speeds up the time milk or other food empties from the stomach). As a result vomiting reduced but the battles over feeding became increasingly more intense as the amount of milk Cassie took dropped lower. Around four months of age it was suspected the cause of her vomiting and feeding refusal was due to milk protein allergy or intolerance and her formula was switched to a hypoallergenic formula. And still she continued to reject feeds. Only now, things were worse.

She now screamed when placed into a feeding position. After two days of almost complete feeding refusal Cassie was admitted to hospital. A number of diagnostic tests returned negative results. In hospital the nurses taught Amanda how to force Cassie to feed. Because Cassie did not show signs of hunger, Amanda was advised to feed her every three hours.

I met Cassie two weeks after discharge from the hospital. Amanda wanted help to resolve Cassie's feeding issues. She was emotionally burnt out and could not continue to force Cassie to feed in the way she was taught at the hospital. I asked Amanda to demonstrate how she was instructed to feed Cassie. When it was 'time' for her feed, Amanda laid Cassie on a crib sheet in preparation to swaddle her tightly. Cassie started to scream, wave her arms and kick frantically as soon she realized she was about to be swaddled. Amanda picked up her firmly swaddled baby and held her in a feeding position in her arms. Cassie's head was held in the crook of Amanda's elbow in a vice-like grip that prevented her from turning her head to the side. Cassie was still screaming, so Amanda had no trouble putting the nipple into her mouth. But Cassie did not close her mouth around the nipple, and instead kept screaming. Amanda then maneuvered her hand holding the bottle in a way where she could grip Cassie's cheeks and chin to force her mouth to close around the nipple. She was then able to manipulate Cassie's jaw to move in a way that caused a little milk to be squeezed into her mouth, between muffled screams. By this stage, Amanda had tears streaming down her face. I felt for her and for Cassie but I needed her to continue to demonstrate what she had been taught in order to understand the situation.

Cassie fought hard for about 10 minutes. Then she suddenly went quiet and within seconds appeared to drop off to sleep. Once asleep, she started to rhythmically suck and drained the bottle in five minutes.

When the bottle was empty, Amanda removed it from Cassie's mouth. Within seconds she woke and smiled at her mother.

No wonder Amanda felt she couldn't continue to feed Cassie in this way. As an observer I found this scene disturbing. I could only imagine the stress that both Cassie and Amanda had endured over and over again as a result. Force-feeding served the purpose of making Cassie drink, but this was achieved at a great emotional cost to her, her mother, and no doubt father as well.

What was especially sad in Cassie's case is that the unfortunate sequence that led to forcing her to feed could have been avoided. I asked Amanda how much milk she had been told Cassie needed. She told me. When I calculated this into milliliters (ml) per kilogram (kg) per day, it was a little over 180 ml/kg/day or 3 oz/lb/day, the amount generally recommended for preterm babies before reaching their expected date of birth. Cassie was four months past what had been her expected date of birth. The standard calculation to estimate milk requirements for babies aged three to six months in Australia is 120 ml/kg/day or 2 oz/lb/day. (See Chapter 6 for more on estimating how much milk babies might need.) While this was likely to have been an oversight on her doctor's part, I was surprised that this error had not been identified during her recent hospital admission.

Unbeknown to Amanda, she had been trying to make Cassie drink more than she needed starting from around the time of her expected birth date had she been born at term. And the gap between what Cassie needed and what Amanda tried to make her take widened as Cassie matured. As the gap widened so too did the amount of pressure Amanda needed to exert to make her drink what had become an unrealistic overestimation of her milk requirements. The pressure Amanda exerted caused Cassie to develop an aversion and then reject feeds even when hungry. Cassie screamed and fought feeds because of the stress of being repeatedly forced to eat more than she needed and not due to pain associated with acid reflux.

And she regurgitated large amounts of milk because she was overfed and not because of delayed gastric emptying. There was no family history of allergies and Cassie displayed no signs indicating an allergic response to her milk before being switched to hypoallergenic formula. Gastro-intestinal symptoms believed to be due to milk protein intolerance were likely due overnutrition occurring as a result of overfeeding.

The good news for Cassie and her parents was that the situation was resolved using strategies described in Chapters 9 to 11. Two weeks after Amanda started following the recommended strategies Cassie started to get excited when she realized she was about to be fed and ate well, consuming a realistic amount of milk for her age and weight. She was switched back to a regular formula and all medications were ceased a few weeks later.

No baby should be forced to feed. If a baby is not capable of feeding she requires specialized feeding equipment. If a baby who is physically capable of feeding is not feeding well or drinking enough for healthy growth, this indicates a problem. **Force is not a solution.** It only complicates the situation.

Most of us recognize when we're forcing a baby to feed. However, do you know that many strategies recommended to 'encourage' a baby to continue feeding involve enough pressure to make baby's feeding experience unpleasant, annoying or stressful? It's important to know that certain types of 'encouragement' can cause and reinforce a feeding aversion.

Subtle forms of pressure

You might unknowingly pressure your baby to feed in the following ways:
- **Restraint:** Restraining or restricting baby's head or arm movements so she can't turn her head away or push the bottle away.
- **Placing the nipple into baby's mouth against her wishes:** She might try to avoid feeding by clamping her lips shut or by turning her head, arching back in a tense manner or by pushing the bottle away with her hands or feet, and despite these signs of rejection you place the nipple into her mouth.

- **Inappropriate response to baby's cues:** Not allowing baby to push out the nipple. Or by following baby with the bottle when she's tense and tries to break away by sharply turning her head to the side or arching back. (This is different to a baby leisurely turning her head to look around while continuing to suck.)
- **Trying to make baby suck:** This may be attempted by applying pressure to her cheeks or under her chin.
- **Jiggling and twisting the bottle:** This is usually done in an attempt to get baby to suck. This might trigger a newborn's sucking reflex.
- **Squeezing milk into baby's mouth:** People do this using a soft-sided bottle, syringe or spoon.
- **Trickery:** Getting baby to suck on a pacifier, then slipping it out and the bottle in.
- **Distraction or entertainment:** When baby fusses or becomes upset or stops feeding, parents often resort to methods that aim to distract or entertain their baby, such as standing, rocking, bouncing, singing, walking around, dangling toys, playing videos on their smart phone or tablet for baby while feeding. While these strategies don't apply pressure per se, they are often employed in an attempt to placate a baby while she's being pressured to eat.

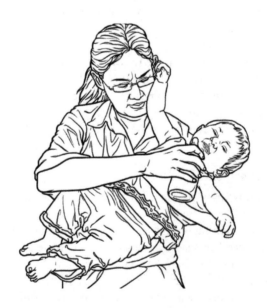

- **Offering repeatedly:** Offering the bottle over and over again when a baby is telling you – by her behavior – that she doesn't want it will at the very least, annoy her. How do you feel being offered food repeatedly after you have said 'no'? At worst, it's a form of harassment, which if repeated at other feeds could cause a feeding aversion. Blaire's story is an example of what can happen when a baby is repeatedly offered feeds over an extended period of time.

Baby Blaire

Blaire would readily take 2 ounces (60 ml) of milk and then refuse. When offered again she would either reject or take a sip or two before rejecting. Her mother Christine would offer her the bottle every five minutes until she either finished the bottle or until two hours had elapsed from the start of her feed. She would try to sneak the bottle into Blaire's mouth while she was held in her arms, while she played with toys, while she was in the bath. In fact, when Blaire was awake Christine was constantly trying to get her to take the bottle. While Christine did not use force, she harassed Blaire with repeated offerings over an extended period of time.

Christine commented that she believed Blaire would starve if it were not for her repeated attempts to feed her. Little did she know that her repeated attempts to feed her were probably the reason Blaire had become averse to feeding. It was certainly the reason Blaire's aversive feeding behavior continued. Once Christine followed the feeding recommendations described in Chapters 9 to 11, Blaire willingly fed at regular intervals throughout the day, and took larger volumes at each feed, sufficient to maintain healthy growth, in less than 10 minutes. Christine could then enjoy fun times with Blaire without feeling she needed to be continually trying to make her feed.

Basically, 'pressure' involves anything a parent or caregiver does to try to make baby continue feeding after she displays signs that she has had enough or is not interested in feeding.

Of course parents could use these strategies under certain circumstances, for example to encourage a sleepy baby to remain awake long enough to feed or support a baby who is too weak or sick to feed, and cause no problems whatsoever. But when such strategies are employed to make a healthy alert baby continue eating more than she wants, it can make the feeding experience unpleasant. Whether such strategies cause a feeding aversion depends on whether it upsets baby or not, and how often it's repeated.

> **The more parents try to control how much their baby eats, the more frustrating and upsetting the situation becomes for everyone involved, and the less incentive baby has to willingly eat.**

What happens when babies are pressured to feed?

As a result of interviewing over 1000 parents who consulted with me regarding an infant bottle-feeding aversion, I discovered a pattern in the progression of babies' aversive feeding behavior, how parents interpret this, and the way infant feeding aversions are managed by health professionals. I describe this below, and also explain why a baby might behave as she does from a developmental and behavioral perspective. My aim is to help you to identify if 'pressure' is the original cause of your baby's aversion and/or something that could be currently reinforcing her oppositional feeding behavior. (Please use a preterm baby's adjusted age.)

Birth to six–eight weeks

A baby can experience **feeding-related** issues at this age, for example sucking problems or dietary self-regulation problems such as overfeeding or underfeeding. But it's unusual for a baby younger than six weeks to get upset as a result of pressure to feed, or display behavior that indicates she has become averse to feeding.

Baby has an active sucking reflex at this age. Triggering her sucking reflex by upwards pressure under her chin or by jiggling the bottle means it's not hard for a parent to make her suck even when she's not hungry. Basically she can't fuss while her sucking reflex is triggered. But she can after the bottle is removed. If she gets more milk than her stomach can comfortably hold she's likely to be unsettled due to discomfort after the feed, and could regurgitate part or most of the feed shortly after feeding or when outside pressure is applied to her stomach eg, by lifting her legs when changing her diaper, while she's seated in a slumped position or laying over a parent's shoulder.

Six to eight weeks

Six to eight weeks is typically the age that parents claim their bottle-fed baby first started to display troubled feeding behavior **during** feeds. At this age, baby's sucking reflex has started to fade. As a result she has more control over the feed than she did at a younger age. She can now stop sucking when she chooses. She might stop because she needs to burp, or to poop or pass gas, or simply to pause before starting again or because her hunger is satisfied. Due to her newfound ability to decide when she's done, she might appear to suddenly take less than she did a few days ago, especially if she was previously overfed.

Baby's satiety cues (described at the start of this chapter) are often overlooked, mostly because parents are unaware of what these behaviors mean. Confused as to why baby is no longer drinking her usual amount, a parent might start to apply gentle pressure to make baby empty the bottle or complete an amount believed to be what she needs. Her sucking reflex has not completely disappeared, and so it's relatively easy to make her continue sucking. Unaware that this is an involuntary response to her sucking reflex being triggered, the parent is then convinced that baby was hungry after all and that they did the right thing making her complete the feed.

Two to three months

As baby matures, her sucking reflex gradually fades. So applying pressure under her chin or jiggling the bottle is now losing effectiveness. It's getting harder to make her finish the bottle if she chooses not to.

Initially, baby's fussiness occurs in direct response to the unpleasantness of being pressured. But when repeatedly pressured to feed, she links feeding with unpleasant or stressful experiences. And she also learns to expect the pressure.

In the early stages of a feeding aversion, baby usually feeds okay at the start of the feed, provided she's hungry, but stops sucking and fusses after consuming **an almost identical amount each time**. This figure varies between babies. As a result of past stressful feeding experiences, she doesn't enjoy feeding and so she's taking just enough to ease hunger pangs.

The parent assumes she stops because she needs to burp. Baby is burped and the bottle reoffered. But she refuses to suck and starts to cry. No pressure has been applied at this point. But past experiences have taught her ... it's coming. While she's held in a feeding position she's tense and upset as she is expecting to be pressured as she has in the past. The parent tries their usual strategies to make baby feed. But baby continues to be upset. The parent tries to placate baby's cries using distraction techniques such as standing, rocking, bouncing, walking, singing, or dangling toys before baby's face as they continue trying to make her eat, with minimal success. Her cries continue to escalate until the parent eventually gives up.

Oblivious to the cause of baby's fussing, the parent wonders if she doesn't like the taste of her formula, and so switches a number of times. Next the parent might suspect that baby is having trouble feeding as a result of the equipment, and tries every bottle and nipple they can find, with fleeting success.

Between two to three months of age, baby learns to link the steps that indicate feeding is about to start. If she has been pressured or forced to feed in the past, as soon as a bib is placed around her neck or when she's laid in a feeding position, she knows something bad is going to happen. She becomes tense, cries, kicks and screams in anticipation.

The parent might try to feed baby in different places such as baby rocker, car seat, or propped on pillows. This usually works initially because baby doesn't associate these places with being pressured to feed. But if she's pressured in these places she soon will, and at that point she rejects feeding in these places as well. Alternatively, the parent might try to trick baby into taking the bottle by giving her a pacifier and once she starts sucking, they slip it out and the nipple in. But this too has limited success.

At a loss to explain baby's distressed behavior, the parent becomes convinced that pain is responsible. Baby is taken to the doctor. Unable to see any physical cause to explain baby's distress, many health professionals, often without asking the parent a single question about how they manage baby's feeds, **assume** the cause is acid reflux. Some **healthy, thriving** babies are misdiagnosed with acid reflux at a younger age owing to milk regurgitation and abdominal discomfort caused by overfeeding, or distress due to sleep deprivation. **The fact that a baby is thriving rules out acid reflux.** If baby was not diagnosed with acid reflux previously, she's highly likely to be diagnosed now, as acid reflux is commonly blamed as the reason for feeding refusal by medicos and others.

Or her doctor might prescribe acid suppressing medications on a trial basis.

Three to four months

By now baby's sucking reflex has completely disappeared and sucking involves a voluntary action. Baby is now able to decide when and if she's going to suck.

With each passing day baby is getting bigger, stronger, more aware, and more capable of resisting her parents' attempts to make her feed. The parent tries every strategy they can think of, eg, trickery, cajoling, distraction, entertainment, to get her to feed without force, unaware that these methods involve a level of pressure that can turn her against feeding and reinforce a feeding aversion. Feeding times might extend to one or two hours each. Ultimately, the parent feels they cannot let things continue as baby will soon need to sleep and so, reluctantly, resort to using more intense means to force baby to feed. Feeding time has now become a battle of wills, and a vicious cycle develops.

Diagram 3.1: Cycle of pressure

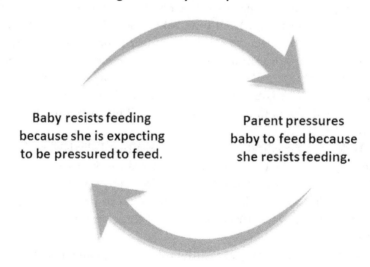

Baby resists feeding because she is expecting to be pressured to feed.

Parent pressures baby to feed because she resists feeding.

As a result of pressure, baby has become averse to feeding and now only willingly eats when seriously hungry and takes less than she needs to support healthy growth. By repeatedly pressuring baby, the parent constantly reminds her that feeding is stressful; so baby keeps trying to avoid it.

At other feeds baby acts like she's confused ('conflicted feeding behavior'). This is because she needs food to relieve the discomfort of hunger, but she doesn't want to feed because she now finds feeding unpleasant or stressful. So she tentatively sucks before pushing away crying, and almost instantly indicates she wants the bottle again, has a couple more sucks and pushes it away again. This is repeated over and over. It appears like she's having trouble staying latched on or that she's pushing away because of pain. The parent restrains her arms to prevent her pushing the bottle away, and holds the nipple firmly in her mouth, resisting her efforts to push the nipple out with her tongue and may try to restrict her head movements to prevent her turning away. But this upsets baby all the more.

As a result of this drawn out feeding process, baby becomes weary. She stops crying, her eyes close and body relaxes as she becomes drowsy. She then starts to rhythmically suck, guzzling the feed in record time.

The parent is concerned that the acid suppressing medications given to baby are not working or that baby's doctor may have overlooked a physical problem. By this age, baby might have been seen by multiple medical specialists and received a number of diagnoses to explain her behavior. Each time baby is seen by a different health professional, or receives a new diagnosis, or is prescribed a different medication, or trialed on new formula, the parent is filled with hope that this might provide a solution, and end the stress the family endures. But hope is usually short-lived. Medications and switching formula will do nothing to resolve a feeding aversion caused by pressure.

Following a medical diagnosis, concern that baby is experiencing pain may cause the parent to remove or reduce pressure on baby to feed, which can have a positive effect on baby's feeding behavior. However, this may not last. If baby continues to drink less than the expected amount, pressure is returned and consequently so does baby's distress.

Between visits to various health professionals, many parents figure out that if they get their baby into a drowsy state first and then slip the nipple into her mouth, she will suck. In a drowsy state, baby is not fully aware of the circumstances, and so her guard is down. She's hungry, and consequently feeds without resistance when drowsy or in light sleep.

Family life revolves around getting baby to sleep, choosing the precise time when she's most likely to suck and carefully feeding her so as not to wake her. Once baby is too deeply asleep, she will no longer suck. So this process is repeated many times throughout the day and night. Some parents might resort to syringe or spoon-feeding milk into baby's mouth with varying degrees of success. But it's a drawn out process of coaxing and cajoling, and one feed blends into the next with brief breaks for naps in between.

If baby's growth is satisfactory, the parent might be advised to 'Keep doing what you're doing' or 'Do whatever you need to do to get X amount of milk into her' by their health professional. If the target amount is not achieved, or if baby's weight gain slows, the parent might be advised to concentrate baby's formula or give high-energy formula, so that she receives more calories in less volume. Or it might be recommended that she be given solid foods starting from four months of age or younger.

Four to five months

It's around this age that an unresolved feeding aversion may start to negatively impact on baby's growth. Concerns about baby's growth make parents feel even more compelled to force baby to feed, the very thing that's causing baby's feeding aversion, and the opposite of what she needs. The whole family is impacted by stress on a daily basis.

Around this age, all the usual medical treatments have been tried and proven unsuccessful. With medical options exhausted, baby's health professionals start to question whether her feeding issues could be behavioral. Baby is referred to a speech or occupational therapist for further assessment. She might be diagnosed with an uncoordinated suck to explain her conflicted feeding behavior, or an oral aversion to explain why she's vigorously opposed to having the nipple in her mouth. But baby knows how to suck; she's choosing not to because she wants to avoid the stress associated with being made to feed against her will. And she's willing to put other things in her mouth. It's just the bottle she wants to avoid. Or it's assumed her distress is due to fear as a result of remembering past painful feeding experiences before medical treatment. But it's not pain she fears, it's being pressured or forced to feed.

The parent **might** be advised to stop trying to force baby to feed. But continues to use gentler forms of pressure believing this encourages baby to eat. Perhaps the parent is advised to shorten the duration of baby's feeds, for example, limit feeds to a maximum of 30 minutes.

But five seconds of pressure is five seconds too long. The parent now pressures baby with less intensity over a shorter period of time, but the result is the same. Any pressure will reinforce baby's aversive behavior, and so nothing improves.

By now the parent has lost faith that health professionals will provide a solution, and searches the internet every spare minute looking for answers.

Five to six months

The situation continues to spiral downwards. It's getting harder to feed baby during sleep now. Due to increased brain development her ability to perceive her surroundings during light sleep is enhanced and she's more easily awoken. Growth has become a serious concern: baby might be lean or classified as 'failure to thrive'. Baby's doctor tells parents if the situation doesn't improve she may need a feeding tube.

Desperate to spare her from tube feedings, and with the hope the situation will improve once she starts to eat sufficient quantities of solid foods to maintain her growth or better, the parent continues the drawn out feeding rituals, unaware that by doing so they're reinforcing baby's feeding aversion.

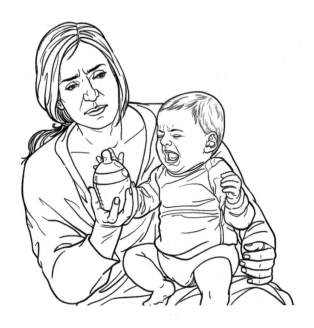

Six months and over

Once feeding becomes a battle of wills, there is no winner. An adult who is bigger and stronger might overpower a baby and make her take more than she's willing to take and thus win the battle, but by doing so, lose the war because they reinforce baby's feeding aversion.

By this stage even baby's health professionals are admitting defeat. Their attempts to resolve baby's aversion to bottle feeding have proven ineffective. The focus now rests on getting baby to eat enough solid foods to make up for the loss of calories she should be getting from milk. If successful this will maintain her growth until she's old enough to stop bottle-feeding and drink sufficient fluids from a cup.

Unfortunately, an unresolved bottle-feeding aversion increases the risk that baby could develop an aversion to eating solid foods. When a parent is reliant on baby eating sufficient quantities of solids to maintain her growth, there's a good chance that she's going to be pressured to eat. Similar to bottle-feeding, pressure to eat solids occurs in various forms and degrees. Gentler forms of pressure are typically viewed as encouragement.

If a baby is repeatedly pressured to eat more solids than she's willing to eat, or if the experience of eating solids is often upsetting, she could develop an aversion to solids (regardless of whether she's averse to bottle-feeding or not). More specifically, she's not averse to solid foods but rather displays aversive behavior trying to avoid the unpleasant or stressful feeding experiences that occur as a result of being pressured or forced to eat against her will. If she does develop an aversion to eating solids, meal times become yet another nightmare for baby and her parents. Feeling defeated, physically and emotionally drained, most parents will at this point start to consider tube feeding as a source of relief.

While this path is common, not all babies who develop a feeding aversion will follow the same path and those who do won't necessarily do so at the listed ages. Only a small percentage of babies with unresolved feeding aversions end up with feeding tubes.

Diagram 3.2 Downwards spiral of pressure-induced feeding aversion

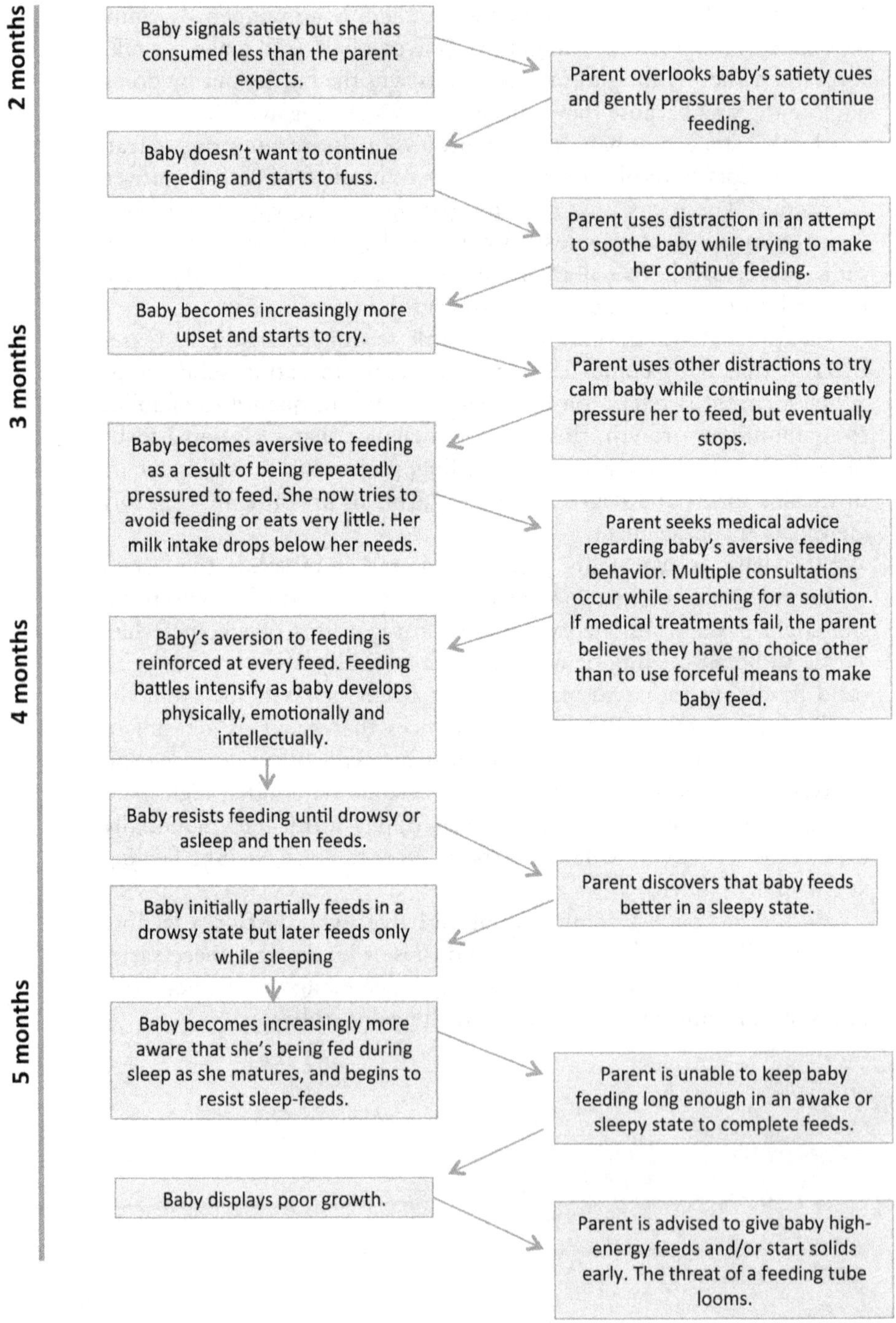

2 months

Baby signals satiety but she has consumed less than the parent expects.

Parent overlooks baby's satiety cues and gently pressures her to continue feeding.

Baby doesn't want to continue feeding and starts to fuss.

Parent uses distraction in an attempt to soothe baby while trying to make her continue feeding.

3 months

Baby becomes increasingly more upset and starts to cry.

Parent uses other distractions to try calm baby while continuing to gently pressure her to feed, but eventually stops.

Baby becomes aversive to feeding as a result of being repeatedly pressured to feed. She now tries to avoid feeding or eats very little. Her milk intake drops below her needs.

Parent seeks medical advice regarding baby's aversive feeding behavior. Multiple consultations occur while searching for a solution. If medical treatments fail, the parent believes they have no choice other than to use forceful means to make baby feed.

4 months

Baby's aversion to feeding is reinforced at every feed. Feeding battles intensify as baby develops physically, emotionally and intellectually.

Baby resists feeding until drowsy or asleep and then feeds.

Parent discovers that baby feeds better in a sleepy state.

Baby initially partially feeds in a drowsy state but later feeds only while sleeping

5 months

Baby becomes increasingly more aware that she's being fed during sleep as she matures, and begins to resist sleep-feeds.

Parent is unable to keep baby feeding long enough in an awake or sleepy state to complete feeds.

Baby displays poor growth.

Parent is advised to give baby high-energy feeds and/or start solids early. The threat of a feeding tube looms.

Why babies feed during sleep

Many babies who have become averse to bottle-feeding will feed when drowsy or during light sleep. Parents learn they cannot pressure baby to feed while she's sleeping if they are to avoid waking her. They know there's little chance of getting her to eat if she was to awaken. So they're mindful to back off at the slightest sign of resistance (something they also need to do when feeding baby while she's awake).

By feeding during sleep, baby avoids the stress associated with being pressured or forced to feed. In a drowsy or sleepy state, she is not fully aware she's being fed, and therefore she's not on edge in anticipation of being pressured, like she is when fed while awake. In a drowsy or sleepy state, a hungry baby's guard is down, sucking instincts kick in, and she feeds well.

The reasons for sleep-feeding vary depending on whether parents feed baby once she's **already asleep** (often referred to as 'dream feeding') or if baby **falls asleep while feeding**. Making this distinction will be important when it comes to solving your baby's feeding aversion.

Feeding baby when already asleep

Sleep-feeding is often recommended to parents as a way to avoid the stress of feeding a strongly resistant baby. Alternatively, parents attempt sleep-feeds at night as a way to increase baby's milk intake and discover by chance that their baby sucks well without resistance when drowsy or asleep.

Encouraged by reduced stress levels for baby (and parent), and increased milk intake while sleep-feeding, many parents begin to feed their baby at each nap. The more milk baby receives in a sleepy state, the more she resists feeding while awake. And so it's not long before sleep-feeding becomes the **only** way some babies feed.

Feeding during sleep provides relief for baby and parents. But **it doesn't provide a solution to a baby's feeding aversion.** It's an extremely restrictive and exhausting process for parents, but most continue to provide sleep-feeds because they know of no other way to get their baby to feed.

Falling asleep while feeding

A baby who has become averse to feeding might fall asleep **while feeding** for a number of reasons, and suck in a drowsy state, including:

- **Exhaustion as a result of fighting feeding:** Tiredness is a common reason why babies **without** feeding aversions fall asleep while feeding. But babies who are averse to feeding are hyper-vigilant and very tense at feeding times. A baby who is averse to feeding might fall asleep while feeding if she becomes worn out after a prolonged battle of wills. As she becomes drowsy, she then starts to suck.
- **Feeding-sleep association:** Some babies fall asleep while feeding because they learn to rely on feeding as a way to fall asleep. Baby then wants to feed when tired and ready to sleep. She sucks well while drowsy, releasing the nipple once deeply asleep. (For further explanation of sleep associations see Chapter 12.)
- **Psychological response to avoid stress:** A small percentage of babies who are averse to feeding fall asleep while feeding when they're powerless to lower their stress levels any other way. After a prolonged battle, resisting her parent's efforts to make her feed, baby goes quiet, her eyes glaze over, she falls asleep and then sucks well, eating quickly. As soon as the bottle is removed from her mouth she wakes and is happy.

Why pressure is often overlooked as a cause

While many health professionals – including pediatricians, midwives, pediatric nurses, child health nurses, speech and language pathologists, occupational therapists and pediatric dietitians – work closely with babies and parents, it doesn't mean they're knowledgeable about infant behavioral problems, like feeding aversion due to pressure. I have had many such health professionals as clients regarding **their** baby's behavioral feeding aversion. Jenna, a UK pediatrician, commented 'We're not taught about behavioral problems.' After resolving his son's behavioral feeding aversion, Jonathan, a USA pediatrician, commented 'I think this experience has made me a better doctor. I now realize that not all baby problems have a medical cause.'

Doctors in general, including pediatricians and pediatric specialists, are not trained to identify **behavioral** causes for infant crying or feeding and sleeping problems that commonly trouble physically well babies.

Not even the most experienced professor in pediatric gastroenterology or neonatology will be proficient in infant feeding management or experienced in recognizing behavioral feeding problems. While most doctors learn the basics, behavioral feeding and sleeping problems are generally not something that's within their area of expertise.

Pamela relayed her doctor's comments 'Let's hope there's a physical cause. If Harper has developed a feeding aversion due to psychological reasons it's much harder to resolve.' While her doctor may not have known how to resolve a feeding aversion to due psychological (behavioral) reasons, at least he was aware that there are reasons beyond medical causes for babies to become averse to feeding.

Even when health professionals are aware of behavioral reasons for babies to become averse to feeding, most don't provide sufficient time during consultations to pinpoint the cause, let alone explain to parents how to resolve this highly complex problem. Time restraints may limit the consultation to physically examining baby, making a diagnosis based on the parents' description of baby's distress at feeding times, writing a prescription and escorting parents to the door.

> **Lack of awareness of behavioral causes means a physical cause is typically blamed for aversive feeding behavior.**

Even after many years specializing in infant and toddler feeding problems, assessment and explanation regarding a feeding aversion takes me around 90 minutes. This is because I send clients a preformatted questionnaire consisting of over 80 questions about their baby, her birth, health, growth, feeding equipment, feeding patterns and behavior, sleeping patterns and behavior and parents' infant feeding practices, which is answered and returned to me before we speak. If I had to verbally ask these questions, the process would take well over two hours. A proper diagnosis takes time.

Before describing solutions to an infant bottle-feeding aversion caused by pressure, we need to address the elephant in the room – the possibility of a physical problem. It's highly likely that your baby has already been diagnosed with a medical condition, or two or three, to explain her aversive feeding behavior. If not, you're probably worried about a physical problem. So the next step is to rule out pain and physical causes.

4
Rule out medical problems

> It breaks my heart seeing Ethan in pain and not being able to help him. So far we have taken him to three different doctors. He's been on four medications and we have switched his formula three times. He's now on a hypoallergenic formula. Nothing seems to be helping. I am so worried that he's suffering because of a physical problem that the doctors have overlooked. – Belinda

Like most parents who are confronted by the stark reality of an infant feeding aversion, Belinda suspects her baby's troubles are due to pain because of a physical problem. I observed Ethan feeding. While he was indeed distressed at feeding times, his behavior at other times did not indicate that pain was responsible for his distress. Belinda later commented that Ethan was a happy baby except when feeding, and that he slept well. This would not be the case if he had a physical problem causing pain.

Babies who become averse to feeding often display distressed behavior at feeding times that can appear like pain.

While pain is one of the **least likely** reasons for **healthy** babies to develop an aversion to bottle-feeding, it's by far the **most frequently blamed cause.** As a potential cause, it needs to be assessed.

If you're worried – like most parents – that your baby's feeding troubles are due to a physical problem or medical condition that's making it painful for him to feed, getting the diagnosis right is your number one priority! **You** can tell if your baby's distressed behavior is due to pain, and if he has a physical problem. You just need to know what signs to look for.

My experience: medical problems are seldom the cause

Most babies I see in regards to a bottle-feeding aversion are not in pain, nor do they have a medical condition. Yet 98 percent of feeding aversion cases I am involved with had been diagnosed with acid reflux and treated with one or multiple medications. Forty percent were diagnosed with milk allergy or intolerance and switched to hypoallergenic formula – usually after medications to treat acid reflux failed to make a difference to baby's feeding behavior. Shockingly, in the majority of cases, parents reported that their baby had no observable physical signs or behaviors consistent with these conditions! That is, besides feeding refusal and poor growth: both of which also occur with behavioral feeding aversions. After I described the various ways babies are pressured to feed, 100 percent of parents admitted that they had been repeatedly pressuring their baby because they were worried about their baby's milk intake or growth.

Parents usually only consult with me regarding an infant feeding problem once they've exhausted medical options. So I am not implying that medical conditions such as acid reflux, milk protein allergy and others don't exist. Or that these conditions can't cause babies to become averse to feeding. I'm simply pointing out that misdiagnosis of the cause of infant feeding aversion is disturbingly common.

Your task at this point is to determine whether your baby's distressed feeding behavior occurs because it's painful to feed or due to other reasons.

Pain is unlikely to be the cause if

It's relatively easy to **rule out** pain as the cause of a baby's distressed or conflicted feeding behavior by assessing how he responds in other circumstances. Pain is **unlikely** to be responsible if...

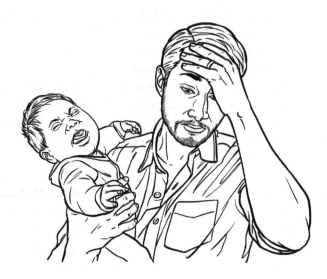

... baby is happy when you stop feeding him

If baby is happy as soon as you stop trying to feed him pain is probably not the cause of his feeding problems. Pain fades; it doesn't suddenly disappear just because the feed has ended.

... baby is content between feeds

If baby is content between feeds, feeding refusal is probably not due to pain. Discomfort associated with acid reflux, milk protein allergy or intolerance, or chronic constipation is **not** restricted to feeding times. Your baby would be distressed at random times day and night in addition to feeding times if he's suffering pain due to a physical problem.

... baby feeds well in certain situations

If baby predictably feeds well in certain situations, for example during the night or while drowsy or asleep you can probably rule out pain. If pain was responsible for distress while feeding during the day or while awake, you'd expect him to also experience pain while feeding at night or when sleep-feeding.

If you're still worried

Whether your baby displays behavior that means pain is unlikely or not, you may still be worried about a physical cause. So your next task is to determine if he displays any signs or symptoms that point to a physical problem. You might be thinking 'Surely this is something best left to his doctor?' Yes and no. Read on to understand why I recommend that you check.

Physical conditions that cause pain

A number of conditions can make it painful or difficult for a baby to suck, swallow or feed, these include:

- acid reflux (also called gastro-esophageal reflux disease or GERD)
- milk protein allergy
- gastro-paresis (delayed gastric emptying)
- constipation
- mouth ulcers
- **severe** oral thrush
- teething
- tongue tie.

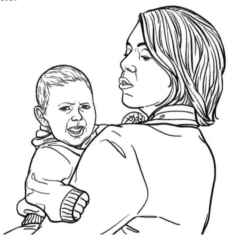

Signs and symptoms

These conditions have **clearly observable physical signs and behavioral symptoms.** As your baby's caregiver, you can see any physical signs as readily as your doctor can during a routine medical examination. He/she might be able to see into baby's throat better than you, but that's not where physical signs will be evident for **most** of the conditions diagnosed as a reason for feeding aversion. And you're better placed to identify behavioral symptoms than a doctor. Table 4.1 describes the signs and symptoms associated with commonly diagnosed conditions.

Table 4.1: Physical conditions – signs and symptoms

Condition	Symptoms	Evidence needed to prove responsibility	Signs that indicate this condition is unlikely
Acid reflux Incidence of GERD is estimated at 1:300[1]	• Distressed behavior at all feeds. • Prolonged periods of inconsolable screaming separate from feeding both day and night. • Regurgitation of bloodstained milk. • Poor sleep. • Poor growth or weight loss.	• Presence of associated symptoms. • Relief of symptoms and infant distress within two weeks following treatment. • Inflammation or ulceration of baby's esophagus seen via gastric scope. **Note:** It is not possible for a doctor to confirm a diagnosis of acid reflux during a routine examination.	• Absence of associated symptoms. • Baby feeds well in sleepy state. • Baby calms quickly once the feed has ended. • Baby is relatively content between feeds.

Milk protein allergy		
Incidence 1:50 formula-fed babies.[2] 1:200 babies receiving only breast milk.[3]	• Presence of symptoms indicating an allergic reaction. • Timing of symptoms coincides with the introduction of milk proteins into baby's diet. • Inflammation of baby's intestinal tract confirmed by rectal scope or Calprotectin stool test. • Disappearance of symptoms within two weeks of the elimination of milk proteins from baby's diet. **Note**: Allergic symptoms can also be seen with airborne and contact allergens.	• Absence of symptoms indicating an allergic reaction. • Formula-fed baby has been on same formula for longer than one month without symptoms. Breastfeeding mother's diet is unchanged and baby is over one month of age.

• Vomiting.
• Diarrhea.
• Blood and mucous in stools.
• Signs of allergic reaction such as coughing, sneezing, wheezing, runny nose, rashes or eczema.
• Distressed behavior at all feeds.
• Irritability due to abdominal discomfort.
• Poor sleep.
• Poor growth or weight loss.
• Anaphylaxis.

Note: Most affected babies display allergic symptoms before one month of age, often within one week after the introduction of cows' milk based infant formula.[4]

Condition	Symptoms	Evidence needed to prove responsibility	Signs that indicate this condition is unlikely
Milk intolerance Incidence is estimated at 5 to 15 per cent.[5]	• Diarrhea. • Bloating. • Extreme flatulence. • Infant distress due to intestinal spasms. • Fussy feeding behavior or refusal. • Poor growth or weight loss.	• Presence of symptoms. • Disappearance of symptoms once baby's formula is switched to a hypoallergenic formula. **Note**: Tests for lactose intolerance are unreliable in infants. False positive results will occur due to transient lactase insufficiency (aka lactose overload) which is associated with overnutrition.	• Absence of gastro-intestinal symptoms. If gastro-intestinal symptoms are present and baby's weight gains are good, assess the possibility of lactose overload. (See Chapter 5).
Gastro-paresis Incidence unknown	• Vomiting. • Excessive belching. • Bloating – abdomen looks distended. • Poor appetite. • Fussy feeding behavior or refusal. • Poor growth or weight loss.	• Gastric emptying study. • Barium swallow.	• Healthy growth. • If GI symptoms are present assess the possibility of overfeeding. (See Chapter 5.)

Constipation	<ul><li>Hard, dry, pebbly stools.</li><li>Straining.</li><li>Distress at random times due to abdominal discomfort.</li><li>Reduced appetite.</li><li>Fussy feeding behavior or refusal.</li></ul>	Diagnosis is based on appearance of hard dry pebbly stools. **Note**: Random, brief episodes of constipation would be an unlikely cause of feeding aversion.	• Soft or watery bowel motions.
Mouth ulcers	<ul><li>Ulcers visible on gums, tongue, inside cheeks or roof of mouth.</li><li>Fussy feeding behavior or refusal.</li></ul>	Ulcers are clearly visible inside baby's mouth.	Absence of ulcers.
Oral thrush	<ul><li>White patches on baby's tongue, gums, inside cheeks, roof of mouth or back of throat.</li><li>Mouth ulcers.</li></ul>	Visible presence of mouth ulcers accompanied by white patches inside baby's mouth.	Absence of visible signs or presence of mild thrush without ulceration. **Note**: Oral thrush, unlike thrush on a baby's bottom, is seldom painful. It would need to be very severe, to the point of ulceration, to prevent a baby from feeding.

Condition	Symptoms	Evidence needed to prove responsibility	Signs that indicate this condition is unlikely
Teething	• A new tooth visible at gum surface. • Swollen gum. • Blood blister on gum. • Fussy feeding behavior or refusal. • Fussing between feeds. • Poor sleep.	Visible signs of tooth about to erupt or already erupting through gum surface.	No visible signs of tooth or swollen gums. **Note:** Teething discomfort rarely lasts long enough to cause a feeding aversion.
Tongue tie Tongue tie does not cause pain but tongue tie snip can.	• Uncoordinated sucking pattern. • Milk leakage from mouth while feeding. • Sucking problems will be evident from the time of birth. **Note:** A tongue tie is more likely to impact on a baby's ability to breastfeed than bottle-feed.	• Visible evidence of tongue tie when examined by a health professional. • Improvement in feeding following tongue tie snip (frenectomy).	• History of sucking well from a bottle. • Baby sucks well while in a drowsy or sleepy state.

If your baby displays any unusual signs that might indicate illness or a physical problem, or if you're worried that your baby is suffering from pain due to a medical condition, have him examined by a doctor.

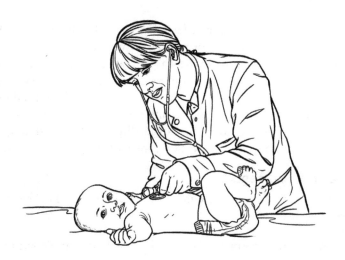

Treatments

A doctor might prescribe or recommend a number of treatments to alleviate discomfort or pain associated with these conditions. These include:

- **Acid suppressing medications** such as a H2 receptor blocker (eg, Ranitidine and Famotidine) or a proton pump inhibitor (eg, Omeprazole, Lansoprazole and Esomeprazole) may be prescribed to treat acid reflux.
- **Prokinetic agents** (eg, Domperidone, Metoclopramide, Bethanechol or Erythromycin) may be prescribed to treat gastro-paresis as these medications make the stomach empty faster and thereby reduce regurgitation of stomach contents (reflux).
- **Hypoallergenic infant formula** may be recommended to treat suspected cows' milk protein and soy protein allergy or intolerance.
- **Aperients,** also called laxatives, may be recommended to treat constipation.
- **Mild local anesthetic gels** may be recommended to numb the sensation of discomfort caused by mouth ulcers.

- **Analgesics**, aka painkillers, may be suggested to alleviate discomfort believed to be caused by teething.
- **Antifungal** medications may be recommended as a treatment for an oral thrush infection.

Note: Medications and hypoallergenic formula **don't cure** these conditions; rather they relieve or minimize symptoms caused by them. Effective treatment, which in the case of acid reflux, milk protein allergy or intolerance and gastro-paresis may need to be continued over the long term, will alleviate pain associated with these conditions. Therefore, pain will no longer reinforce baby's aversive feeding behavior and his fear and avoidance of feeding will fade and disappear within a matter of days to two weeks ... **provided pain is the cause.**

Why medical treatments fail

Your baby's feeding aversion might continue despite medical treatment for three reasons:

1. **Ineffective treatment:** The condition remains and continues to cause pain.

2. **Combined causes:** When pain passes, either naturally or because of effective treatment, baby's feeding aversion may continue because he has been repeatedly pressured to feed or because of another reason listed in Chapter 1.

3. **Misdiagnosis:** If baby displays no signs or symptoms associated with the diagnosed problem, he may have been misdiagnosed.

If your baby is one of a small percentage of babies afflicted by a medical condition, don't assume it's the cause of his feeding aversion, and thus ignore other possibilities. A medical condition won't spare him from developing a behavioral feeding aversion. In fact, it **increases the risk** if his refusal to eat due to discomfort caused by a medical condition is met with pressure.

Misdiagnosis: acid reflux and milk allergy or intolerance

Misdiagnosis of acid reflux and milk allergy or milk intolerance as causes of infant feeding aversion, and many other behavioral baby care problems that cause infant distress, is widespread in western societies.

I asked Mark, an Australian pediatric gastroenterologist, why he thought babies are so often diagnosed with acid reflux and milk protein allergy to explain aversive feeding behavior. He replied, 'Of course, we assume that behavioral reasons have been assessed prior to a patient being referred to us. Our job is to diagnose or rule out organic (physical) causes.' I wonder how many health professionals assume that someone else has already assessed and ruled out behavioral causes when this has not been the case?

Medical doctors are trained to diagnose **medical conditions**, and that's what they do. Often without asking the parent about their infant feeding practices, in particular whether they're pressuring their baby to feed, and in many instances without observable physical signs or behavioral symptoms that point to the diagnosed condition.

A diagnosis of acid reflux and milk allergy or intolerance may be **based solely** on the parent's perception that a baby's distressed or conflicted feeding behavior is due to pain. Or because acid reflux and milk protein allergy are two common **physical** reasons for babies to experience pain while feeding. Or based on other mistaken assumptions, such as these:

TRUE OR FALSE?

1. Acid reflux is a common cause of feeding aversion.

FALSE: While acid reflux can cause a feeding aversion, it's rare for normal, healthy babies to suffer from acid reflux. But alarmingly common for healthy babies to be misdiagnosed with acid reflux during brief consultations, simply because the reason for crying, sleep disturbance or feeding refusal is not understood.

2. Back arching is a sign of acid reflux.

FALSE: Sandifer's syndrome where a baby turns his head to the side and writhes in pain is associated with acid reflux. Back arching does not provide evidence of acid reflux. Normal healthy babies will turn their head or arch back to distance themselves from something they want to avoid. Babies troubled by a feeding aversion due to any reason, the most common being pressure, will arch back to prevent their parent from putting the nipple in their mouth or to try to break away from the bottle. They do so to avoid a situation they have learned is unpleasant or stressful.

3. When a baby will only feed while sleeping this points to acid reflux.

FALSE: Sleep does not desensitize a baby to pain. If pain is responsible for a baby's aversive feeding behavior while awake, then pain would cause baby to wake and cry in distress when sleep-feeding is attempted. (Why babies who are averse to bottle-feeding suck well during sleep is explained in Chapter 3.)

4. Blood in stools provides proof of milk protein allergy or sensitivity.

MAYBE: Blood in stools is commonly associated with milk protein allergy or intolerance. But blood in stools can be due to other causes, for example, an intestinal infection, and 'nonspecific colitis' (meaning the cause is unknown). Streaks or spots of blood on stools may be due to a tiny tear on the inside of baby's anus due to passing constipated stools, or due to lactose overload, which causes acidic stools that burn baby's anus and bottom.

5. Babies are often sensitive to foods eaten by breastfeeding mothers.

FALSE: If your bottle-fed baby receives breast milk, you may be relieved to learn that most mothers can eat what they like without impacting their babies. The incidence of babies reacting to foods eaten by the mother is believed to be 1:200. Without any abnormal gastro-intestinal signs like frequent, explosive bowel motions, mucous or blood in stools, it's highly unlikely baby is reacting to foods eaten by the mother. In cases where there are abnormal GI signs, these are far more likely to be related to lactose overload (explained in Chapter 5) which is a common breastfeeding problem that occurs when a mother has an oversupply of breast milk. In the case of a thriving bottle-fed baby, overfeeding/overnutrition is a common reason for abnormal GI symptoms, such as vomiting and frequent foul smelling stools, whether baby receives breast milk or formula.

6. Babies are too young to develop behavioral problems

FALSE: Many people assume 'behavioral' implies a child is acting in a naughty or manipulative way. And because babies can't behave in these ways, they don't consider the possibility of behavioral problems. 'Behavioral' does not imply a baby is behaving in a deliberately difficult manner.

Babies experience behavioral problems. In fact, behavioral problems are the most common reasons for physically well babies to become distressed and to experience feeding and sleeping problems. For example, aversive feeding behavior due to being pressured to feed (see Chapter 3), overfeeding, which causes gastro-intestinal symptoms, is a behavioral problem linked to feeding management (see Chapter 5), and a sleep association problem, which causes broken sleep and distress due to sleep deprivation, is a behavioral problem related to how baby is settled to sleep (see Chapter 12).

Babies are young but they can think, feel and remember according to their stage of development. I've encountered a number of cases of babies as young as seven weeks with behavioral feeding aversion. In fact, this is around the age when problematic behavior in response to being pressured to feed first becomes apparent.

Beware of the internet! It's rife with misinformation about the signs of acid reflux. Just about everything a baby does – for example, crying when put down, throwing up milk or not throwing up milk in which case it's claimed to be 'silent reflux', eating more often than expected supposedly to soothe the pain, refusing to eat allegedly because it's painful to eat, poking out his tongue, hiccups, wet burps and belching – are often claimed to be symptoms of acid reflux. Similarly, there's a lot of misinformation about milk allergy or intolerance.

Unfortunately, misinformation is not exclusive to the internet. It's also spread by health professionals and people in general.

When you read or hear false claims from a number of different sources, you start to believe they're true.

The Medical Maze

When **behavioral** causes and solutions for infant feeding aversion are either unknown or overlooked by parents and health professionals, an assessment of potential causes is **limited** to medical causes and solutions.

When this happens countless babies troubled by a feeding aversion and their parents become trapped in the Medical Maze for months or years – attending numerous medical and allied health appointments, trialing different infant formulas, multiple medications and dosage changes, and undertaking a battery of diagnostic tests.

As you can see, on the next page, there are multiple combinations of medications and formula changes that could be trialed. **No amount of medications or dietary changes will make a difference to a behavioral feeding aversion.** If the cause of your baby's aversion to feeding is behavioral then searching for a medical solution will prove fruitless.

Medication and formula changes

Some health professionals prescribe medications and recommend dietary changes using a 'Let's try this and see if it helps' approach, seemingly believing it won't hurt to try. But it can! This can further complicate a baby's feeding aversion, and needlessly so in cases where baby has no physical signs that point to the diagnosed condition.

If your baby is diagnosed with a medical condition, check for signs associated with the condition or ask his doctor to provide testing or proof. Don't just put him on bitter tasting medications or hypoallergenic formula based on a guess, or out of desperation. And don't overlook the possibility of a behavioral feeding aversion occurring as a result of being pressured to feed (explained in Chapter 3).

Diagram 4.1: The Medical Maze

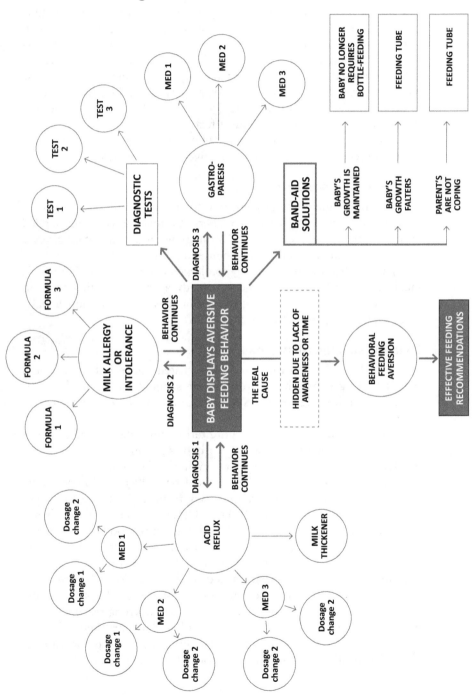

Acid suppressing medications: side effects

The side effects of acid suppressing medication can or may include headache, nausea, vomiting, diarrhea, constipation, stomach pain, intestinal cramping and others.[9] A number of secondary adverse effects are also associated with changing the natural acid balance within baby's intestinal tract as a result of acid suppressing medications. These include increased risk of food allergy, respiratory and gastro-intestinal infections.[10] The more medications given to a baby, and the higher the dosage, the greater the risk of side effects.

Many babies require force to take bitter tasting medications, which has the potential to contribute to aversive feeding behavior.

Hypoallergenic formula: side effects

If a baby is allergic to the proteins in milk, then hypoallergenic formula is necessary. However, when hypoallergenic formula is recommended as a 'Let's try it and see if it helps' strategy without signs of an allergic reaction it could have unintended consequences.

The unpleasant flavor of hypoallergenic formula won't provide much incentive for a baby who is already averse to feeding to want to eat. However, if hypoallergenic formula is the only food a baby receives, he will eventually drink it.

Band-Aid solutions to maintain growth

If the medications and dietary changes listed above fail to resolve a baby's feeding issues, health professionals might recommend one or more of the following strategies to maintain or improve his growth.

- **Thickened feeds:** AR (anti-regurgitation) formula, adding cereal or a food thickener to breast milk or baby's formula.
- **High-energy feeds:** Regular strength formula provides 20 kilocalorie (kcal) **per ounce (67 kcal per 100 ml)**. Commercially produced high-energy formulas vary from 22 kcal to 30 kcal per ounce (75 to 100 kcal per 100 ml). Other ways parents are advised to increase energy content is by adding extra scoops of powdered formula, or oils (eg, MTC oil), or carbohydrates (eg, maltodextrin) to baby's formula or to breast milk. (**Note:** Do not increase the energy content of your baby's feeds without his doctor's permission as this could have serious and potentially life-threatening consequences if not done correctly or for the wrong reasons.)
- **Start solids early:** Many parents are advised to start their babies on solids at an early age (before four months of age) to compensate for reduced calories as a result of a bottle-feeding aversion.

- **Appetite stimulant:** Certain antihistamine medications, such Cyproheptadine (Periactin®), can increase hunger and may be prescribed in the hope of increasing baby' desire to feed.
- **Feeding tube:** A feeding tube is **usually**, but not always, used as a last resort after medical treatments to fix baby's feeding aversion have failed or if his growth is seriously compromised.

I call these 'Band-Aid' solutions because while they're recommended to compensate for poor growth occurring as a consequence of an **unresolved** feeding aversion, they **do nothing** to correct the underlying cause of a baby's aversive feeding behavior.

They can be helpful when babies have **physical** problems that prevent them from feeding well, or for babies with reduced sensitivity to hunger cues, but they're not always successful in resolving growth problems in the case of feeding aversion, **because they don't address the cause.**

When a baby is averse to feeding, what usually happens as a consequence of increasing the energy (calorie/kilojoule) content of his milk feeds or by giving him solids at an early age is that he gets more calories/kilojoules in his belly and as a result drinks even less milk or avoids bottle-feeding for longer periods.

A feeding tube – which prevents a baby from self-regulating his dietary intake (deciding how much to eat), and in many cases removes incentive to feed orally and denies opportunities to develop oro-motor skills – opens the door for a gamut of potential problems down the track. The best solution is to resolve baby's aversion to bottle-feeding; something that is **not** achieved with Band-Aid solutions.

The further a situation is removed from what is natural, the greater the risk of complications. I have seen many **behavioral** feeding aversion cases where the baby was given two or three different prescribed acid suppressing medications **at the same time,** and one or two prokinetic medications, plus high-energy, thickened, hypoallergenic formula and solids. This tangled web of potential drug side effects and other complications makes it even more challenging to figure out the 'cause and effect' of baby's aversive feeding behavior.

Response to failed treatment

Some families are trapped in the Medical Maze for so long that they exhaust all medical options. Others opt out sooner and search the internet for other potential causes. Either way, at some point as a result of failed treatment the focus turns away from finding a medical solution. It's then suspected that baby's aversive feeding behavior occurs or continues as a result of one of the following problems:

- a psychological response to the memory of painful feeding experiences or
- a sucking problem (see Chapter 2)
- a sensory processing disorder (described in Chapter 1) or
- a behavioral or psychological problem due to 'unknown cause'. (Unknown because 'pressure' – described in Chapter 3 – is not considered.)

And so baby may be referred to an allied health professional such as a speech and language pathologist (SLP), occupational therapist or pediatric dietitian, where an effective solution may or may not be provided. To be effective, a solution must address the cause!

It's not just doctors who misdiagnose acid reflux, milk allergy and milk intolerance because they don't understand the cause of a baby's troubled feeding behavior. I have had numerous parents relay that various health professionals, such as pediatric and child health nurses, speech and language pathologists, occupational therapists, dietitians, naturopaths and other parents, have blamed one of the medical reasons described in this chapter. And so baby might be sent back to his doctor where he's referred onto yet another medical specialist for more tests, medications and formula changes. All the while the true source of his distressed feeding may continue to be overlooked and therefore reinforced.

Other parents may be told that their baby's aversive feeding behavior is due to his temperament or that he simply doesn't like feeding. Neither statement is correct. All babies are capable of enjoying feeding. While some babies are more sensitive and therefore more easily upset than others, distress at feeding time indicates a problem.

Psychological response to pain

> Liam has been on acid reflux medications for two months. It hasn't helped. The doctor thinks he has developed an aversion to feeding because of remembering the pain and even though it's no longer painful he's afraid to eat because he thinks it will cause him pain. What can I do to help him get over his fear that bottle-feeding will be painful? – Samantha

If despite treatment a baby's oppositional feeding behavior continues, some parents are told this is because their baby remembers the pain he experienced while feeding before treatment. While it's possible for aversive feeding behavior to continue for a **short time** after pain has been removed, **the memory of pain** doesn't cause aversive behavior to continue over the long term. Remember, behavior must be reinforced to continue. If there's no pain, then a feeding aversion due to pain is no longer reinforced.

Have you ever had really bad food poisoning, and when you encounter that food again you turn away because the mere thought of eating it makes you nauseated? This is an example of a physical event causing an aversion. If despite these feelings you ate this food again and suffered no ill effects, then your aversion would lessen. It continues to fade with repeated uneventful events until you're completely over your aversion. Similarly, when baby experiences multiple feedings with no pain, then his fear of pain while feeding **disappears within days** and so too does his aversive behavior.

Samantha waited for months for Liam's aversive behavior to resolve. But Liam didn't suffer from acid reflux. His feeding aversion occurred because he was pressured to feed. While waiting for 'the memory of pain' to fade, Samantha had continued to pressure him to feed; hence why Liam's behavior continued.

Escape the maze!

If your health professional has overlooked 'pressure' as a potential cause of your baby's feeding aversion, then you need to consider it. It could free you from the Medical Maze, save you time, money, and most important of all your baby's health and wellbeing.

Regardless of whether your baby's troubles first began as a result of a physical problem such as acid reflux or milk protein allergy, or being pressured to feed, or another reason described in Chapter 1, it's likely that he is currently pressured to feed in subtle or obvious ways. It's also possible that pressure is the **only** thing now reinforcing his behavior.

Before I explain how to resolve a baby's feeding aversion that is reinforced by pressure, you need to identify mistakes – yours or your health professional's – that might be have caused you to feel you needed to pressure him to eat. If you don't, it might prevent you from resolving his feeding aversion and you may face similar feeding problems with any future baby you have, for the same reasons.

Parents feel duty-bound to make sure their baby eats for numerous reasons. These fall into different categories based on the following mistakes:

- **Mistake 1:** Belief that parents must control how much baby eats. (Explained in Chapter 5.)
- **Mistake 2:** Overestimating baby's milk needs. (Explained in Chapter 6.)
- **Mistake 3:** Unrealistic expectations regarding baby's growth. (Explained in Chapter 7.)
- **Mistake 4:** Assuming baby is not eating enough because he's not eating or gaining as much as expected. (Explained in Chapter 7.)

In the next chapter we look at your role when feeding your baby. Understanding this can help relieve the pressure **you feel** when feeding your baby, and may help break the cycle of feeding aversion.

PART B:
Correct misperceptions

5
Know your role

> Ava (aged 8 weeks) doesn't demand feeds. She
> doesn't show hunger like other babies. Even after
> sleeping for 6 hours straight at night she doesn't
> wake hungry. I feed her every 3 hours. She will
> take 2 ounces in 5 minutes and then act like that's
> enough. But it's not enough. It can take me 30
> minutes to an hour to get her to take the rest of
> her bottle. I'm sure she would starve if I didn't
> make her drink. – Fiona

It's unclear whether Ava has developed a feeding aversion based on
Fiona's description. I am concerned that she could head down that
path. I observe Fiona feeding Ava and confirm that the wheels that
lead to a feeding aversion are indeed in motion. Ava accepts the bottle,
but right from the start of the feed Fiona constantly prompts her to
keep sucking by jiggling the bottle. When Ava stops after drinking two
ounces, Fiona tries to make her continue by manipulating her jaw. Ava
is getting very upset, so Fiona stops and tries to burp her. Ava calms
when the bottle is removed and she's sat up but cries as soon as Fiona
lays her back to continue the feed.

Fiona is making a number of common errors. She's not giving Ava long enough to demand feeds, not letting her set the pace of the feed, and she's not letting Ava decide when she's done. Instead Fiona is trying to control when, how much and how fast Ava eats. If she keeps this up, Ava's feeding behavior and milk intake could get worse. So I explain to Fiona her and Ava's responsibilities in the feeding relationship and how to interpret Ava's behavioral cues. This is the topic of this chapter.

Mistake 1: Believing parents must control how much baby eats

Trying to make a baby feed when she doesn't want to is not fun. It can be as stressful for parents as it is for babies. So why do some do it? Parents pressure their babies to feed out of loving concern. They worry that their baby might not sleep, become dehydrated, fail to gain sufficient weight, become unwell or die if they don't make sure their baby consumes what they believe or have been told is a minimum amount of milk. In cases where a baby has developed a feeding aversion, parents pressure or force their baby to feed because they're not aware of how to remedy the situation.

Many parents are taught to believe they must control how much their baby eats, either by health professionals or family members. This might be necessary in **unusual** circumstances, such as a baby who is incapable of eating enough for healthy growth due to a physical or neurological problem. But it's **not** the case for normal healthy babies and children who are physically able to eat. Most healthy babies are capable of deciding how much they need to eat.

The belief that a parent must control how much a healthy bottle-fed baby drinks is flawed. Consider this. Breastfeeding is the biological feeding norm for a baby and you cannot control how much a breast-fed baby drinks, right? So why would you need to control how much a bottle-fed baby drinks? I appreciate why parents might believe this in the case of infant feeding aversion, because their baby refuses to eat enough, but it's still flawed thinking none the less.

Regardless of the reasons or intentions, trying to control how much a baby eats can have the opposite of the desired effect.

> **Trying to make a baby or child eat against her will is THE MOST effective way to turn her off feeding and eating.**

A healthy baby might require **support** while feeding, but she doesn't need others to **control** how much she eats.

Can babies self-regulate food intake?

While babies cannot get their own food, and they're not able to make healthy food choices, they can self-regulate their **intake** – decide when and how much they need to eat. Babies and children are sensitive to the energy (calories or kilojoule) content of food and can therefore regulate meal size and meal times.

Neurologically normal babies are born with energy regulation capabilities. In simple terms that means they can decide how much food their body needs to support healthy growth according to their genetically determined size and shape. This is not something they need to learn or think about. It's already programmed into their subconscious brain by the time of birth.

Finely tuned mechanisms in baby's brain and body help her respond to changing conditions to maintain an internal state of balance or harmony. These enable her to recognize when she's hungry and decide when to stop eating. They take into account energy variations in the food she eats, her growth rate, her metabolism and energy expenditure related to activity, and control her appetite. For example, when her blood sugar level drops below a certain point her body releases hormones that cause discomfort due to hunger. The sensation of fullness as her stomach expands tells her when to stop eating. And the feeling of satisfaction as the digestion of fat and protein occur in her intestinal tract carries her through until the next time her body needs food.

To self-regulate the amount of milk taken from a bottle, a baby needs to have the ability to:

1. signal hunger
2. suck effectively for as long as required to receive sufficient nutrients
3. stop when she's had enough, plus ...
4. she has to want to eat.

All baby needs to do to self-regulate her intake to meet her growth and energy needs is to follow her internal sensations of hunger and satisfaction. Not all babies are physically capable of signaling hunger and/or consuming enough for healthy growth, for example preterm babies, sick babies, babies with neurological impairment, or babies who have problems sucking effectively.

When baby is averse to feeding

In the case of feeding aversion, baby **lacks the desire** to eat. She will ignore her internal cues of hunger until she is ravenous and she will break away from the feed before reaching satisfaction. She does this because she finds the experience of feeding while awake to be upsetting or stressful, and not because she's **incapable** of knowing how much her body needs.

I will explain how to resolve her feeding aversion starting from Chapter 9, but first I would like you to understand more about your baby's self-regulation capabilities and your responsibilities when feeding her. This may help you feel more at ease following my feeding rules and recommendations.

Your responsibilities when feeding your baby

You are the key to resolving your baby's feeding aversion. To prevent or resolve an infant feeding aversion you need to stick to your role when feeding your baby. Canadian dietitian, Ellyn Satter coined the term 'Division of Responsibility' to define the parent and child's roles in relation to feeding.[11]

Division of Responsibility
- The parent is responsible for what.
- The child is responsible for how much (and everything else).

Regardless of the reasons you may have started to pressure your baby to eat, you need to stop. **You're not responsible for how much she eats.** That's your baby's responsibility. You do however have certain responsibilities when it comes to feeding her, which differ depending on her physical abilities. Let's clarify your responsibilities when feeding your baby.

Your responsibilities include:

- Offer feeds when baby signals hunger, or if she's a non-demanding baby, offer at regular intervals appropriate for her stage of development.
- Select suitable feeding equipment that allows her to easily access the milk at a pace she can comfortably handle (ie, not too slow or fast). And feed her in a position that enables her to suck effectively. (See Chapter 2.)
- Feed her in an environment that helps her to remain attentive to feeding.
- Observe her behavior as she feeds. If she fusses, you need to figure out what's troubling her and respond accordingly.
- End the feed when she signals she has had enough.

Your baby's responsibility is to decide if she will accept what you offer and how much she will drink. You should **not** pressure, coerce, cajole, distract or try to trick her to make her accept the bottle or drink more than she's willing to drink.

You may also need to support her so that she can effectively feed to satisfaction. How much support a baby requires at feeding times depends on her level of maturity.

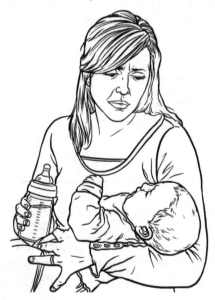

How much support do babies need?

A healthy baby's ability to self-regulate her dietary intake varies according to her stage of development. And so too does the level of support required from caregivers. Table 5.1 matches age with dietary self-regulation abilities.

Table 5.1: Dietary regulation ability for age

	Signal hunger	Suck effectively	Signal satiety
Preterm (before reaching expected date of birth)	Nil or limited capacity	Nil or limited capacity	Nil or limited capacity
Birth to 2 months	Capable	Capable	Limited capacity
Over 2 months	Capable	Capable	Capable

Note: A baby's capabilities could vary from the table above depending on her health and physical abilities.

Preterm baby

Prior to 36 weeks gestation, preterm babies in general can't self-regulate their milk intake. They don't give clear signals of hunger. They are awake for only brief periods of time. They have a weak or non-existent suck and tire quickly while feeding. By necessity, health professionals involved in baby's care while in a special care nursery will decide, what, when, and how much milk she consumes. Nurses will employ feeding methods that ensure she receives a predetermined amount. Once discharged from hospital, baby's parents take over feeding responsibilities.

From around 36 weeks gestation, most neurologically and physically healthy preterm babies can **signal hunger** and **suck effectively**. Many babies born before 36 weeks achieve similar skills around the time they reach 36 weeks gestation, but not all. Some do so at a later stage. Others who were born extremely premature or who experienced complications as a result of their prematurity or congenital disabilities could experience difficulties feeding and require additional support over the long term.

Provided a baby has no major health issues affecting her sucking ability, around the time of what would have been her expected date of birth her ability to self-regulate her dietary intake will be similar to term babies of the same age. Please use 'adjusted age' – the age she would now be had she been born at her expected due date – when considering a preterm baby's self-regulation skills from this point. Subtract the number of weeks she was born early from her **actual** age to work out her **adjusted** age.

Birth to three months

Normal healthy full term babies, and preterm babies once they reach their expected date of birth, have the ability to signal hunger, and they're strong enough to feed with a little support from parents.

At this age babies' sucking reflex is present. A reflex is an automatic, involuntary response. The sucking reflex is triggered by pressure on the top of a baby's tongue and roof of her mouth by her mother's nipple, nipple of a bottle, pacifier, her fingers or a parent's finger. The sucking reflex is strong at birth, fades over time and disappears completely between three to four months of age.

In the early weeks a baby has limited ability to control the flow rate from a bottle and signal when she's had enough while her sucking reflex is triggered. But by around six to eight weeks of age she can signal satiety (that is, her hunger is satisfied) and stop sucking when she's had enough.

Hunger cues

From birth to three months her hunger cues include:

- licking or smacking her lips
- sucking on her lip, tongue, fingers, or fist
- fidgeting
- bobbing her head forward and side to side with an open mouth
- opening her mouth wide when touched on the chin, cheek or lips
- fussing and crying.

Note: Be aware that newborns will behave in this way for reasons other than hunger. So you may also need to consider the context, for example the size and timing of baby's previous feed. This will help you determine if hunger is the most likely reason for these behaviors.

Satiety (satisfaction) cues

From birth to three months her satiety cues include:

- sucking slows and stops
- relaxed jaw
- releasing the nipple
- closed lips
- turning her head away
- looking settled and relaxed
- arms and legs are stretched out
- falling asleep.

Over three months

At this age a healthy baby's sucking reflex has disappeared and she can self-regulate her dietary intake to match her growth and energy needs. She can signal hunger, suck effectively with minimal support, and she can signal satiety and stop when she wants to stop.

By now, her memory has increased and she has developed greater skills to communicate than she did at a younger age. She will let you know if she's not satisfied with the amount of milk she's getting and if she's not happy about the response she receives to her behavioral cues while feeding (and at other times). She will express frustration and anger, by fussing, crying, screaming and thrashing body movements if her hunger or satiety cues are overlooked or if something annoys or troubles her while feeding. She will object and robustly resist if you try to make her accept a feed if she does not want to eat or if you try to make her drink more than she wants. And resist with increased intensity as she becomes bigger, stronger and more aware.

Hunger cues

Over three months her hunger cues include:

- fussing or crying
- becoming excited at the sight of the bottle
- leaning towards or reaching for the bottle
- opening her mouth to accept the nipple
- sucking vigorously once the nipple is in her mouth.

Satiety (satisfaction) cues
Over three months her satiety cues include:

- stops sucking
- chews on the nipple or moves it around her mouth
- pushes the nipple out of her mouth with her tongue
- clamps her mouth shut
- turns her head away from the bottle
- pushes the bottle away.

If your baby has not proven she can self-regulate her milk intake by this age, it may be because you have not given her the chance. Or she may be experiencing dietary self-regulation problems.

In summary, infant feeding practices, such as when and how you offer feeds to a preterm baby differ from a newborn and differ again from how to feed a baby over the age of three months. If you don't adapt your feeding practices to match your baby's advancing development, this could mean you unintentionally frustrate her or create unpleasant or stressful feeding experiences that can cause her to become averse to feeding.

Dietary self-regulation problems

Even though a baby may be physically capable of self-regulating her milk intake according to her needs, whether she does so is reliant on receiving appropriate support from her caregivers. Preterm and newborn babies are especially vulnerable to self-regulation problems such as underfeeding and overfeeding.

Underfeeding

Common reasons why a baby might not eat enough for healthy growth include:

1. **Breastfeeding problems:** Latch problems are common in the newborn period. Rarely is low milk supply an issue in the early weeks.

2. **Rigid feeding schedules:** The parent might disregard baby's hunger cues while attempting to make her feed at predetermined times.

3. **Unsuitable feeding equipment:** A baby could tire before completing the feed because of equipment problems; eg, the nipple is too slow,

or the nipple ring is screwed down too tightly on a non-vented bottle, both of which can increase the effort required for a baby to feed. (See Chapter 2.)

4. **Sleep deprivation:** If a baby is not getting enough sleep she might tire and give up or fall asleep before completing feeds. (See Chapter 12)

5. **Feeding aversion:** When a baby has become averse to feeding, she might ignore internal hunger cues because her determination to avoid the stress associated feeding battles is stronger than her need to soothe her hungry belly ... to a point. She will feed when famished but eat only a little. Or she might feed while in a drowsy state or sleeping because she's not aware she's being fed and thus not feeling stressed.

Less common reasons include:

6. **Physical problems:** For example, functional, structural or neurological problems affecting baby's ability to suck; digestive disorders causing discomfort while feeding; illness affecting appetite; or cardiac and lung conditions causing her to tire before she has eaten enough. Most of these problems are identified soon after birth.

How can you tell if your baby is underfeeding? She will initially become very irritable, whine, demand constant attention and cry if she's not receiving sufficient nutrients. (She will do the same if she's not getting enough sleep.) If the problem causing underfeeding persists she will have infrequent bowel motions and gain weight poorly or lose weight. As her body tries to conserve energy she will sleep for unusually long periods and become listless and non-demanding when awake.

Overfeeding

Overfeeding is a far more common problem in developed countries compared to underfeeding. But underfeeding is a more serious problem.

When a baby drinks in excess of what is expected, parents usually question this. However, in many instances overfeeding is overlooked by health professionals, and parents are erroneously told, 'Don't worry,

You can't overfeed a baby.' But this is simply not true. Newborn babies are vulnerable to overfeeding for the following reasons:

1. **Misreading baby's hunger clues:** Most newborn babies have a strong desire to suck that extends beyond the time they need to feed. They like to suck when tired, upset, uncomfortable and for pleasure. They will fuss or cry for many of the same reasons. When baby's fussing and desire to suck are automatically assumed to be due to hunger, this means she might be offered feeds at times when she's not hungry.

2. **An active sucking reflex:** When a baby's sucking reflex is triggered, sucking occurs as an automatic involuntary response. Baby will suck even when she's not hungry. Milk pooling in the back of her throat triggers her swallowing reflex and so she may appear to hungrily guzzle down the feed irrespective of whether she's hungry or not.

3. **Speed-feeding:** It takes time to feel the sensation of satisfaction that follows a meal in both adults and babies. If the flow rate through the nipple is too fast, a baby could feed too quickly and is at increased risk of overfeeding. (See Chapter 2 for the ideal feeding duration for age.)

4. **Pressure:** It's not hard to make a newborn eat more than she wants. You just apply pressure in an upward direction under her chin, jiggle the bottle, or manipulate her jaw movements to trigger her sucking reflex. Many parents do these things to 'encourage' their baby to finish the bottle, unaware that they may actually be pressuring their baby to continue feeding. For a newborn baby this can contribute to overfeeding.

5. **Feeding-sleep association:** If a baby regularly falls asleep while feeding, feeding can become a sleep association. When a baby has learned to rely on feeding as a way to fall asleep she will appear hungry whenever she's tired and ready to sleep. She may also want to feed as a way to return to sleep if her sleep is broken. A feeding-sleep association also makes it difficult for a parent to tell the difference between baby's hunger and tiredness cues.

When a baby overfeeds this **does not** necessarily translate into large weight gains, though it can. Our bodies have thousands of mechanisms that act automatically to maintain a state of balance or harmony within. A baby's internal homeostatic mechanisms will act in ways that reduce or eliminate the effect of overfeeding. And by doing so reduce the risk that she will accumulate excess stores of body fat. The effects of two homeostatic mechanisms are visible. They are:

1. milk regurgitation (reflux)

2. larger or more frequent bowel motions

Milk regurgitation (reflux)

There are limits on how much a baby's stomach can hold. If her stomach becomes overextended by large volume feeds or small frequent feeds provided before the previous feed has emptied from her stomach, she might regurgitate milk; ranging from small spit ups to large forceful vomits.

Larger or more frequent bowel motions

Immaturity of baby's digestive tract means she has a limited ability to produce digestive enzymes, such as lactase necessary to break down lactose. While a healthy baby produces enough digestive enzymes to support healthy growth, her intestinal tract might not be able to digest an **excess** of nutrients that occurs as a result of overfeeding. If nutrients cannot be digested (broken down by digestive enzymes) they cannot enter her blood stream and therefore cannot be stored as body fat. Undigested nutrients will pass through baby's intestinal tract and be pooped out. However, this **does not** occur in a passive way. Baby will display further signs of her body's attempts to digest the excess of lactose (aka lactose overload).

Lactose overload

Lactose overload, also known as transient lactase insufficiency, is a common problem experienced by newborn babies. Lactose overload is not a condition. It's a **feeding management problem**, which causes newborns to display gastro-intestinal (GI) symptoms, such as frequent watery stools when fed breast milk or sloppy foul-smelling stools when fed infant formula. Other symptoms include, bloating and extreme flatulence due to fermentation of lactose in the large bowel. Stools become acidic, which can burn baby's bottom if left too long on unprotected skin. When severe or prolonged, lactose overload can cause blood speckled stools and mucous. Behavioral symptoms include irritability, crying and sleep disturbance due to painful intestinal contractions. Stool samples may provide **false positive** results when tested for lactose intolerance.

There's nothing wrong with healthy babies' ability to digest **normal** amounts of lactose. GI symptoms occur when their intestinal tracts become swamped by **excessive** amounts of lactose as a result of overfeeding in the case of bottle-fed babies (and oversupply syndrome in the case of breast-fed babies).

Lactose-free infant formulas, which include soy and hypoallergenic formulas, relieve GI symptoms linked to lactose overload because baby is no longer exposed to excessive amounts of lactose. However, these formulas are **not** necessary. Preventing overfeeding by addressing the causes of overfeeding will relieve GI symptoms.

When dietary self-regulation problems are overlooked

When parents observe baby's discomfort and GI symptoms most will seek medical advice. But as already explained, because baby is not gaining excessive weight health professionals in general tend to **overlook overfeeding** and so they don't ask how much, how often or how quickly baby is eating, or ask parents about their infant feeding practices. Instead the symptoms associated with overfeeding are typically blamed on conditions such as colic, acid reflux, milk allergy or intolerance, or delayed gastric emptying.

In western societies in particular, normal, albeit distressed, infant behavior due to sleep association problems (see chapter 12) and feeding problems, such as overfeeding, underfeeding and feeding aversion, are **often** erroneously attributed to medical conditions. Parents in general don't receive education from health professionals on how to adapt their infant feeding practices to support their baby to self-regulate her dietary intake, or advice on how to modify their infant settling practices in ways that enable baby to receive the amount of sleep her little body needs. Instead, babies receive a medical diagnosis – or two or three – anti-colic remedies or medications, antacids or acid suppressing medications, prokinetic medications, lactose-fee formula, soy infant formula, hypoallergenic formula, anti-regurgitation (AR) formula, cereal or other milk thickening agent added to baby's formula.

Some medical treatments may **appear** to help in the case of **overfeeding** because they hinder or inhibit a baby's homeostatic mechanisms from functioning as they should. For example, baby might not regurgitate as much milk as a result of medications or thickened feeds, and she might not experience as much gas and her stools might not be as loose or frequent as a result of switching to a lactose-free, soy or hypoallergenic formula (which inadvertently eliminates the symptoms of lactose overload). While **some of the symptoms** associated with overfeeding may be treated in these ways, the **cause** of these symptoms – overfeeding – is not. Failure to address the cause means **other symptoms may continue despite treatment.** As a result, baby might receive multiple diagnoses, numerous medications and dosage adjustments, and dietary changes.

In cases of **underfeeding**, increasing the energy (calories or kilojoules) of a baby's feeds might help improve baby's growth. But without addressing the causes of underfeeding, maintaining baby's growth may continue to be a constant battle. Parents will feel inclined to pressure their baby to take a little more and so the likelihood of a feeding aversion is high.

The second most common mistake linked to infant feeding aversion involves overestimating baby's milk requirements. Read on to discover how this happens.

6
Understand baby's milk needs

> Henry (aged 4 months) weighs 14 pounds 7 ounces (6550 grams). His doctor said he needs to drink at least 25 ounces (740 ml) a day. I have to force him to drink. He often falls asleep during the feed and then drinks better but I can only get him to take 15 ounces (445 ml) maximum. I'm so worried that he's not going to grow properly if he doesn't drink enough. – Emma

While I disagree with parents being told how much their baby 'needs' or 'must have', 25 ounces seems like a conservative estimation of milk volume for a baby of Henry's age and size. I investigate further and discover that Emma is adding extra scoops of formula plus rice cereal into his bottles on the advice of his doctor. The combination increases the energy content of his feeds by a massive 80 percent. This means Emma has been trying to force Henry to consume an excessive number of calories for a baby of his age and size.

It no longer surprises me when parents relay poor advice provided by health professionals about bottle-fed babies' milk volumes. It's an all too common occurrence in the feeding aversion cases I see.

I believe that overestimation of formula requirements, or in Henry's case, caloric requirements, by health professionals or parents, is a major cause of infant bottle-feeding aversion. (Other reasons why parents pressure their babies to feed are explained in Chapters 5, 7 and 8).

Explaining to parents the cause and solution to their baby's feeding aversion is usually not enough to resolve the problem. Some parents need to adjust their expectations about their baby's milk needs. If not, they may feel compelled to continue pressuring their baby to consume unrealistic volumes of milk. Emma didn't need to adjust her expectations about the volume of milk Henry **might** take, but she needed to stop adding extra scoops of formula and rice cereal to his feeds, and resolve his aversion to feeding.

If you have unrealistic expectations about your baby's milk requirements or expected weight gains, you might not know it. Please read this chapter before following my feeding recommendations. Having **realistic** expectations about the volume of milk your baby **might** require is crucial in order to successfully resolve his feeding aversion.

Mistake 2: Overestimating baby's milk needs

Some parents are told their baby requires more milk than he or she actually needs. Of the cases I have been involved with, around 25 percent of parents were quoted amounts by their health professional that were higher, and in some cases as much as 50 percent more, than average for age and weight. Or the health professional failed to take into account extra calories provided by concentrated formula, fortified breast milk, high-energy formula, or additives such as oils, cereal or carbohydrates when estimating milk requirements.

In another 25 percent of cases, health professionals – though using standard calculations – failed to consider the baby's individual pattern of growth. In particular that baby was likely to go through a period of **catch-down** growth as a result of laying down large stores of body fat in the womb or due to overfeeding in the early months. A baby who is undergoing catch-down growth will consume less than the standard amount of milk because he's gaining weight at a slower than average rate. (Catch-down growth is explained in Chapter 7.)

Overestimation of milk requirements is not limited to health professionals. Many parents turn to the internet or the side of the formula can for information on how much milk baby 'should' have, without understanding the numerous reasons why a baby might require less than indicated.

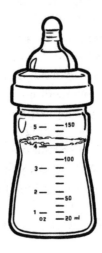

How much milk does a baby need?

Babies come in all shapes and sizes. Their growth patterns differ and so too does the volume of milk **each** baby needs. There are general guidelines designed to provide an **estimation** of how much a baby might need. But these are not appropriate for **all** babies. General guidelines should **not** be used as benchmark figures required by all babies.

General guidelines

When estimating a baby's milk requirements many health professionals use standard figures based on the baby's age and weight. However, it might surprise you to learn that there appears to be no consensus on what these figures should be. The figures differ between countries – and in some instances between health authorities within the same country! The table on the next page compares standard figures commonly used in Australia, USA and the UK.

Table: 6.1: Formula calculations according to country

Age	Australia: NHMRC Infant Feeding Guidelines. Information for Health Workers 2012[1]	USA: The Merck Manual[2]	UK: UK Health Guide to Bottle-feeding 2011
Preterm to expected birth date	180 ml/kg/day 3 oz/lb/day	180–200 ml/kg/day 3–3.5 oz/lb/day	150–200 ml/ kg/day 2.5–3.5 oz/lb/ day[3]
5 days to 3 months	150–200 ml/ day 2.5–3 oz/lb/day	150 ml/kg/day 2.5 oz/lb/day	
3–6 months	120 ml/kg/day 2 oz/lb/day		
7–12 months	90–100 ml/kg/ day 1.3–1.5 oz/lb/day	100 ml/kg/day 1.5 oz/lb/day	500–600ml/ day[4] 17–20 oz/day

Note: These figures are based on regular strength breast milk or infant formula, which is 20 kcal per ounce or 67 kcal per 100 ml. They are estimations and not 'must have' amounts.

Did you notice that the USA recommends 25 percent more and UK recommends 25 to 40 percent more milk for babies aged three to six months compared to Australia? Why the difference? Who knows! A baby would not require 25 to 40 percent more or less calories because his family moved from one country to another.

I favor the Australian figures, especially for babies aged three to six months. Not because I am Australian, but rather because babies' rate of growth naturally slows as they mature. Therefore, it makes sense that babies would require less milk **in relation to body weight** as they mature. However, Australian figures will not apply to every baby. No country's figures will.

Calculations used to estimate babies' milk needs are simplistically based on **age and weight**. At best they provide a rough estimation of what a bottle-fed baby **might** need. At worst they can be way off the mark, and cause parents undue anxiety when their baby doesn't drink the estimated amount. The parent might then disregard their baby's satiety cues and attempt to pressure him to drink more than he actually needs. Repeatedly doing this can cause him to develop a feeding aversion.

Calculations based on age and weight should **never** be quoted as 'must have' or 'should have' amounts for any baby. Finn's story provides an example of just how wrong standard calculations can be.

Baby Finn

Finn lived in USA. At four months of age his weight was 18 lb 4 oz (8280 g) and his length 25 inches (63.5 cm). When comparing weight to length, this meant he was in the overweight category. He was born chubby, weighing 10 lb 2 oz (4600 g) but average length. Plus he had been forced to drink large volumes of milk in the early months, possibly more than he needed as the amount was calculated based on his chubby weight, which included extra rolls of body fat. As he got older and stronger he resisted his mother's efforts to force him to feed. Owing to repeated feeding battles, Finn developed an aversion to bottle-feeding.

After resolving his feeding aversion, Finn was allowed to decide how much he wanted to drink. His milk intake varied, but averaged around 27 ounces per day (800 ml) or around 1.5 oz/lb/day (100 ml/kg/day). This amount was significantly less than USA recommendations of 2.5 oz/lb/day (150 ml/kg/day) for his age, which would have amounted to a massive 45.5 oz (1350 ml) per day based on his weight. It was also lower than Australia's more conservative recommendations for babies aged three to six months. Despite drinking less than his mother and doctor expected, Finn displayed signs of a well-fed baby (described later in this chapter).

Because Finn was overweight but now allowed to decide how much his body needed according to his appetite, his body would go through a period of catch-down growth. His weight gain would be less than average until his body shape had realigned to his genetically determined path. During the period of catch-down growth his milk intake would likely continue to be lower than his doctor might expect – if basing this on standard calculations for age and weight – while his body converted excess stores of fat into energy. After his body size and shape had returned to his natural path, Finn's weight gains and milk intake might then be closer to average figures for age and weight. But not until then.

Note: Don't restrict an overweight or obese baby's diet. Let him decide how much to eat and avoid sleep-feeding.

A baby might need more or less than the amount estimated by their health professional, or formula manufacturer, or a website for a variety of reasons.

The best feeding advice comes from Canada. Canada's health authorities recommend 'parents should let their baby decide how much to drink, and never pressure baby to take more'.[16]

What influences milk requirements?

As mentioned, standard calculations are based solely on the baby's age and current weight. They do not take into consideration the many variables that might influence an **individual** baby's milk needs, such as:

1. **Gender:** In general boys consume more calories than girls of the same age and size.

2. **Genetic endowment:** Whether baby is genetically inclined (inherited traits from mom and dad) to be long, short, lean, chubby or average.

3. **Body fat:** Whether he's currently underweight, overweight or normal weight.

4. **Rate of growth:** Whether he's experiencing catch-up or catch-down growth following a period of underfeeding/undernutrition or overfeeding/overnutrition, which can occur in the womb or the early months after birth due to dietary self-regulation problems described in Chapter 5. US and UK figures for babies aged three to six months don't take into account that babies' rate of growth is in general slower at this age compared to birth to three months. (You will find more about babies' growth in Chapter 7.)

5. **Metabolic rate:** How fast or slow his body burns energy (calories or kilojoules).

6. **Activity levels:** How active he is.

7. **Appetite fluctuations:** Whether he's going through a growth spurt or plateau in growth (which occur between growth spurts).

8. **State of health:** Whether he's currently ill or has recently been ill.

9. **Milk concentration:** Standard figures are based on milk concentration of 20 kcal per ounce or 67 kcal per 100 milliliters. A **healthy** baby over the age of eight weeks who can self-regulate his dietary intake, will regulate his intake **according to the calories** (energy) content and **not the volume**. The higher the energy content of a baby's milk, the less he needs to drink **over the course of the day**.

10. **Solid foods:** The number of calories he receives from solid foods.

My point is, no health professional can say how much milk your baby 'should have'. They can only guess. How much information they use when guessing will determine how close they are to a realistic figure. If their estimation is based solely on your baby's age and weight (as occurs when using standard figures) without consideration of appetite influencers listed above, the amount estimated could potentially be far removed from the amount your baby actually needs.

Your baby might not drink the amount you or your doctor expects, or what I would estimate. And I tend to be more conservative than most.

When I estimate how much a baby might be drinking after getting over their feeding aversion, at times I've been WAY off the mark, like I was in Ivy's case.

Baby Ivy

Ivy developed a feeding aversion because her mother, Hailey, tried to make her drink the amount of milk her doctor had recommended. As a result of her aversive feeding behavior, the doctors tried all the typical medical treatments without improvement, and a series of diagnostic tests, all of which indicated there was no physical problem. (You have read this before and know the drill by now.)

I met Ivy and Hailey when Ivy was five months of age. She showed extreme aversive feeding behavior. She would start screaming as soon as her mother tried to put a bib around her neck and screamed louder when laid in a feeding position. She completely rejected the bottle. Hailey found that with force she could manage to get her to take only 10 to 13 ounces of 24 kcal per ounce formula (which provides 20 percent more calories than regular formula) each day. Ivy would fiercely fight any attempts to feed her and getting her to take that amount would consume almost all her waking hours. At the time, Ivy's weight and length were on the 25th percentile, which was in keeping with her parents' heights. But she needed to have her feeding aversion fixed so that she could continue to grow well.

After assessing the situation, I thought Ivy's low intake was due to a behavioral feeding aversion. And that once this was resolved, she would eat around the Australian standard amount for a baby of her age and size, give or take a couple of ounces. I estimated around 24 ounces based on 24 kcal formula. So I figured a range of 20 to 28 ounces was a reasonable expectation.

As it turned out I was partially correct. Ivy's aversion to bottle-feeding was behavioral, and it was due to force-feeding, and so it was resolved using my feeding recommendations.

But her milk intake, though now higher, did not increase to the amount I estimated. Ivy would very happily drink between 15 to 17 ounces each day but no more.

I was perplexed. For all intents and purposes she appeared to be over her feeding aversion. Why was she not drinking close to what I expected? I checked everything again. Observed a number of her feeds. Hailey was managing feeds as recommended, tick. Ivy was not showing signs of aversive feeding behavior, tick. Ivy was getting enough sleep, tick. Ivy's feeding pattern was appropriate for her age, tick. Hailey reported Ivy had no physical signs that might indicate illness or a physical problem, tick. What was I missing? With all bases covered I came to the conclusion that Ivy just needed a little more time to get into the swing of drinking larger volumes.

Despite her low intake, Ivy showed signs of being well nourished so I suggested Hailey continue and see what happened over the next week. I felt confident that Ivy's milk intake would increase during that time. A week later, no increase in intake. And surprisingly, Ivy had a good weight gain. Thinking, 'That can't be right', I put her weight gain down to fluctuations in body fluids. Ivy looked great. She was happy and energetic and well hydrated, so I recommended that Hailey continue and see what happened in another week. Surely Ivy's milk intake would have increased by then. The week ended. Same. No increase and Ivy had another good gain. What's going on here? How could she gain so well when eating around two-thirds of what most babies her age and size would eat? All looked good, so I suggested Hailey continue for another week. Next week, the same. No increase but gaining well. I was dumbfounded! But by now it was obvious that Ivy knew what her body needed for healthy growth.

Hailey emailed me from time to time over the next 10 months. Usually at times when Ivy's milk intake dropped lower, sometimes to 13 ounces per day. Mostly this was because she was eating a lot of yogurt and solids or she was unwell.

But Hailey reported that there were also times in between these drops when her milk intake would reach 20 ounces. Through all the ups and downs in Ivy's diet her growth was almost textbook. She consistently remained around the 25th percentile for weight and length.

Hailey was initially worried about Ivy's milk intake, but once she got to see that Ivy was growing healthily on the amount she was eating, she stopped worrying and accepted that Ivy needed less than most other babies.

Ivy was bottle-fed breast milk. It's quite possible that Hailey's milk has a much higher fat content than average. Had Ivy been breastfeeding during this time, Hailey would not have known that she was eating significantly less than her doctor was telling her Ivy needed. If Ivy had been allowed to decide how much she ate from the start, she would not have developed a feeding aversion and Ivy, Hailey, Ivy's dad and other family members could have been spared months of needless stress and worry.

The lesson I learned from Ivy is that while I can try to estimate how much a baby might need taking into account the many variables that affect appetite, I can still be wrong. **Only a baby knows how much his or her body needs.**

Give baby the chance to decide

Healthy babies will take the amount they need to achieve their genetically determined size and shape, **if we give them the chance,** and provided we don't unintentionally place barriers in their path like a feeding aversion or other causes of underfeeding described in Chapter 5.

Countless numbers of breast-fed babies self-regulate their milk intake. Their mothers are not told how much milk they 'should have' at each feed or each day. Healthy babies – irrespective of whether they're breast-fed or bottle-fed – don't require others to decide how much milk they need.

Trust your baby's inborn ability to know how much he needs to eat. Follow his hunger and satiety cues and let his biological needs guide his appetite and caloric intake. At the very least give him the chance to show you what he can do. But don't expect him to self-regulate his intake straight away. He needs to get over his feeding aversion first.

If at any time you're worried whether your baby is eating enough, look for signs that indicate he's well fed.

Signs baby is well fed

As a loving parent you want to know your baby is getting enough to eat. That's understandable. However, making your baby drink the amount your health professional recommends is not the only way to know that your baby's nutritional needs are met. You don't need to rely on markings on the side of baby's bottle to tell if he's drinking enough. Table 6.3 describes physical signs that indicate if a baby is receiving sufficient fluids and nutrients.

Table 6.3: Signs of nutritional status

	Well nourished	Not eating enough	Malnourished
Wet diapers	5 or more disposable diapers per day or 6 or more cloth diapers per day.	Less than 5.	Less than 5.
Bowel motions	Regular bowel motions.	Infrequent stools.	Infrequent, green slimy stools (starvation stools).
Appetite	Demands regular feeds.	Constantly demanding/ fussing, whining due to hunger.	Non-demanding.
Mood after feeds	Appears satisfied following feeds.	Irritable soon after feed has ended. (Note: A sleep-deprived baby will also be constantly irritable.)	Falls asleep before completing feed. (There are also other reasons why babies fall asleep while feeding.)

	Well nourished	Not eating enough	Malnourished
Mood between feeds	Mostly happy except when hungry, tired or bored. (Baby could be cranky if he's sleep deprived.)	Content for only brief periods. Often irritable, clingy and demands constant attention to soothe.	Very sleepy.
Energy	Energetic, interactive, inquisitive.	Listless at times.	Lethargic.
Sleep	Sleeps well. (Baby could sleep poorly due to unrelated sleeping problems.)	Difficult to get to sleep. Often wakeful due to hunger. (The same behavior could occur due to underlying sleeping problem. See Chapter 12).	Difficult to arouse.
Weight gain	Baby is gaining **over time**, but might not gain as expected. (Explained in Chapter 7.)	Baby's weight gain is poor or stagnant.	Baby is not gaining and may be losing weight.

A combination of these signs provides an indication of a baby's nutritional state.

If **after resolving his feeding aversion**, your baby displays signs indicating he's well nourished, there's probably little to worry about. If the signs indicate he's not eating enough, his feeding aversion is probably not yet resolved. But also consider other reasons for underfeeding described in Chapter 5. Trying to make him eat more than he's willing to eat using pressure is not the answer.

In the next chapter I explain how mistaken assumptions made when assessing a baby's growth can put baby on a path to a feeding aversion.

7

Clarify growth expectations

> The health nurse said Abby (aged 4 months) is not gaining enough. She said she should be gaining an ounce (30 g) a day, and that I needed to feed her more. I feel sick with worry knowing she's not growing properly. I have to fight with her to make her drink, which I hate doing but I don't know what else to do. We tried adding an extra scoop of formula to the same amount of water, but she drank less. How do I make her want to drink more? – Rebecca

The health nurse has caused Rebecca to suffer needless anxiety by quoting the average weight gain for a newborn, not a four-month-old. This figure exceeds the amount that most babies gain at this age. The nurse would not have misled Rebecca intentionally; it would have been due to limited understanding about infant growth. Regardless, this mistake has had serious consequences for Abby and her family because it has caused Rebecca to use pressure tactics to try to make Abby drink more. Abby has become so traumatized from repeated feeding battles that she's now refusing to eat, and Rebecca is stricken with anxiety.

It might be comforting to learn that only a small percentage of babies experience **genuine** growth problems (in countries where food is plentiful).

However, mistakes made by health professionals when assessing babies' growth, which cause parents needless anxiety, occur more often than you might expect.

If your baby has a feeding or digestive problem that is having a negative effect on her growth, the earlier this is rectified the better. But it's equally important that your expectations about your baby's growth are realistic. If you were to expect her to gain more than she's genetically programed to gain, this could trigger a chain reaction that eventually leads to her not gaining enough.

Mistake 3: Unrealistic expectations about baby's growth

Growth and feeding aversions are connected in the following ways:

- Parents often pressure their baby because of real or perceived growth concerns, or because they believe they need to in order to prevent poor growth. Being repeatedly pressured to feed can cause a baby to become averse to feeding.
- Many babies troubled by an unresolved feeding aversion will get to the stage where growth becomes negatively impacted.

Seldom do health professionals express concern when a baby gains more than expected, which for some babies could signal overfeeding. Rather, an alarm is raised when a baby gains less than expected.

Concerns about poor growth can become a self-fulfilling prophecy when parents try to control how much their baby eats. If their health professional raises concern that baby is not gaining enough, parents will understandably try to encourage their baby to eat more. In some cases, like Abby's and others, mistakes are made. There was no actual growth problem; only an erroneous perception that baby's weight gain was poor. Regardless of whether growth concerns are valid, or a mistake, baby is likely to be pressured to eat against her will. As a result of being pressured, she develops a feeding aversion. And as a consequence of becoming averse to feeding, she doesn't eat enough for healthy growth and genuinely displays poor growth. Then feeding becomes an ongoing battle of wills.

Why mistakes occur

Monitoring the growth of babies is not an exact science. While infant growth charts represent **typical** growth patterns and tables list **average** weekly weight gain figures, **no chart or table can predict the growth of each individual baby.**

When a baby's growth deviates from a typical pattern or baby gains less than expected, how this is interpreted depends on the health professional's knowledge and experience.

Health professionals **vary considerably** in their ability to assess infant and child growth. Not all receive formal training on how to do this. Instead, they learn from others, which also means they can repeat the mistakes of others. Even experienced health professionals can make rookie mistakes. No doubt I've made a few myself!

Brief consultation times generally only allow enough time to examine baby, pop her on the scales and compare her weight gain against average figures. But not enough time to thoroughly assess the situation.

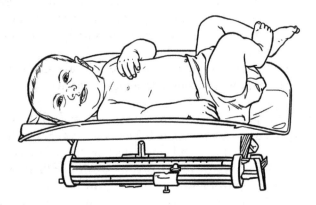

Mistaken assumptions

In the absence of knowledge or information, assumptions are made. The most frequent mistakes regarding infant growth occur as a result of assumptions, for example:

- A typical growth pattern is assumed to be the only normal growth pattern; therefore if baby's weight or length drops to lower percentile curves on an infant growth chart it's assumed she has a growth problem.
- Weight gain within an average range is assumed to be something all babies must achieve; therefore if baby doesn't gain average or expected weight it's assumed this indicates poor growth.

Knowing the number of ounces or grams a baby has gained can be reassuring, but it can also cause needless anxiety if the results are not interpreted within the context of the broader picture. Gaining less than a health professional expects is **not** proof that something is wrong. It just means a **thorough** investigation is necessary. But investigation doesn't occur when assumptions are made.

As a result of these assumptions other reasons for what can **appear like** poor growth, such as variations of normal growth, false alarms or unrealistic expectations, are not considered. And **no assessment** of baby's nutritional state is made to confirm if baby is underfeeding or not.

Variations in normal growth can give a false impression of poor growth. Let's look at these now.

Variations of normal growth mistaken as poor growth

Babies don't all grow in the same way. Not all babies follow a typical growth pattern or gain within an average range for age. There are many variations of normal growth that enable individual babies to achieve their growth potential. Five that are often mistaken as poor growth include:

1. growth plateau

2. breast-fed versus formula-fed

3. natural decline in growth rate

4. catch-down growth and

5. constitutional growth delay.

Growth plateau

Children don't grow in a consistent pattern where every day they're a little taller and heavier than the previous day. Growth occurs in a step-wise pattern. They have growth spurts and plateaus.

A **growth spurt** involves a rapid burst of growth in weight and length that occurs over a matter of days. Growth spurts typically involves increased appetite that last two or three days, but for older babies can last up to a week.

A **plateau in growth** occurs following a growth spurt. Baby eats less than she did during a growth spurt and her weight appears to stagnate or she gains very little for what could be days or weeks. It's typically assumed that baby is gaining less because she's eating less. But in reality she's eating less because her growth has plateaued. Growth plateaus like growth spurts don't last forever. But unlike growth spurts, plateaus in growth can cause unnecessary concern if they are not identified as a normal part of the growth cycle and instead mistaken as poor growth.

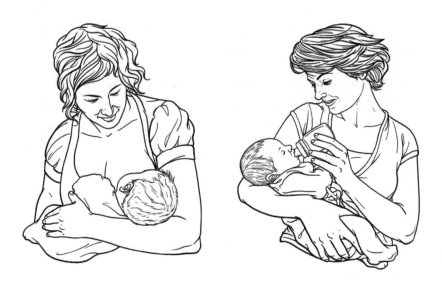

Breast-fed versus formula-fed

In 2006, WHO (World Health Organization) released a series of infant growth charts based on the growth of **breast-fed babies**. These charts demonstrated a noticeable difference when compared against the previously used 2000 CDC (Center of Disease Control) infant growth charts. The CDC charts, while combining data on both breast- and formula-fed babies, largely represented the growth pattern of **formula-fed babies**.

Comparison of WHO and CDC charts demonstrated that breast-fed babies tend to gain more weight in the early months and less after six months compared to formula-fed babies.

Graph 7.1: WHO and CDC male chart comparison[1]

Table 7.1 compares median (average) weight gain figures for age of WHO and CDC infant growth charts.

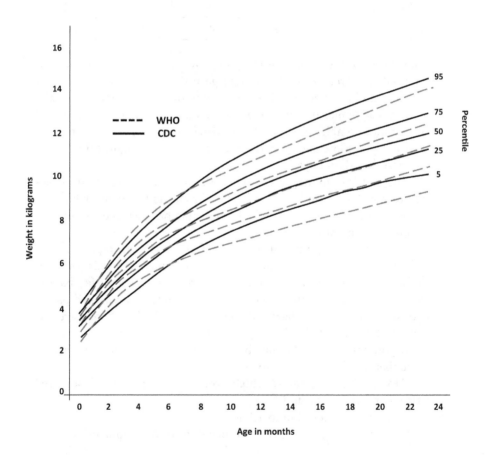

Table 7.1: Median weekly weight gain for age

Age	WHO		CDC	
	Ounces	Grams	Ounces	Grams
2 weeks–3 months	8.5	240	6	175
3–6 months	4.4	125	5.3	150
6–9 months	2.6	75	4	115
9–12 months	1.9	55	2.8	80

Note: These figures represent mid range **over a three-month** period for **male babies**. Average weekly weight gain does not suddenly drop at three-month increments; rather the amount of weight gained gradually decreases as babies mature. 'Average' weight gain is not a pass or fail figure that all babies are expected to reach. Approximately 50 percent of babies gain more and 50 percent less than median figures. In general girls gain less than boys.

There are no infant growth charts that depict the growth of babies who receive breast milk from a bottle. Or charts for babies who start out breastfeeding but are switched to formula before three months, six months, nine months or later.

It's widely accepted that breast-fed babies' growth represents the biological normal growth pattern for babies, but the fact is formula-fed babies don't follow the same growth pattern as breast-fed babies. So while it's not advisable to compare the growth of breast-fed babies against CDC growth charts, it may be unrealistic to compare the growth of formula-fed babies against WHO growth charts.

If you have been told your baby is not gaining within an average range then the first question to ask is:

'Do the figures against which your baby's growth is compared reflect her feeding method?'

And the next question to ask is:

'Are the figures appropriate for her stage of development?'

Natural decline in growth rate

Just like there is no consensus on how much milk babies need, there appears to be no agreement on what is the average amount of weight babies gain. One reason may be that the growth patterns of breast- and formula-fed babies differ. Another is because the average amount of weight gained by babies decreases with age.

It's a common misperception that babies need to gain an ounce (30 g) a day. While some newborns will gain this or more, it doesn't last. As babies mature their rate of growth progressively slows. This is demonstrated by the **curve** of an infant growth chart.

A curve indicates decreased velocity, in this case a gradual decrease or slowing in the rate of growth. If babies were expected to gain weight at the same rate, this would be depicted as a diagonal line on an infant growth chart. Imagine how big a baby would be if she gained an ounce a day for 365 days on top of her birth weight. She would look like a mini sumo wrestler by 12 months!

Table 7.1 also demonstrates that the average amount of weight gained declines – at different rates depending on feeding method – as babies age.

Catch-down growth

After birth the strongest influence on a baby's growth is her genetic endowment (that is the genes her parents have passed to her, whether they're small, thin, tall, large etc). Most people are aware that babies can display **catch-up** growth, which involves accelerated growth after a period of growth delay. Delayed growth can occur in the womb in the case of an intra-uterine growth restricted (IUGR) baby, or as a result of underfeeding in the early months, or due to illness. Fewer people, including health professionals, appear to be aware of **catch-down** growth, also called lag-down growth.

Catch-down growth involves a period of slow growth that is perfectly normal. Babies who display catch-down growth are often, but not always, chubby babies, whose weight sits on a higher percentile curve on an infant growth chart compared to length. Some babies are born with generous rolls of body fat. Others are born proportionate, but much larger than expected given the size of their parents. Others still become chubby in the early months as a result of overfeeding. Because a baby is born large or chubby or becomes chubby in the early months doesn't mean she's destined to remain that way.

At some point, her body will adjust to its genetically determined size and shape. During this time a chubby baby's body will convert extra stores of fat into energy and as a result she gains slowly or her weight might temporarily stagnate, but her growth in length continues at a normal rate. And large but proportionate babies going through catch-down growth may grow at a slower rate for both weight and length compared to others. Baby Ethan provides an example.

Baby Ethan

When Ethan was born his weight was on the 75th and length on the 50th percentile curves of an infant growth chart. Ethan then gained slowly, and his weight and length dropped to lower percentile curves over time. The doctor had told his mother, Gail, it was because Ethan was not getting enough to eat. Gail decided to stop breastfeeding and switch Ethan to bottle-feeding so she could tell how much he was getting and make sure he took the recommended amount. No matter how hard she tried to make him eat, Ethan gained slowly.

By the age of four months his weight and length were on the 20th percentile curve. I asked about Gail's height, which was 5'4", and Ethan's father's height, which was 5'3". This meant that Ethan's length at 20th percentile was in keeping with his genetic endowment. His weight was proportionate to his length. He had a healthy layer of body fat. What Ethan's doctor had mistakenly interpreted as poor growth was in reality catch-down growth.

While there were no growth concerns at that point, Ethan had developed an aversion to feeding as result of being pressured. This situation needed to be resolved so he could maintain his natural growth course. If not, his avoidance of feeding would likely intensify with increased maturity and this could result in poor growth. His feeding aversion was successfully resolved, but I also needed to adjust Gail's expectations about Ethan's growth.

While Ethan was born quite large considering his parents' size, his pattern of growth demonstrated that he was not genetically predisposed to remain large. It was important that Gail recognized this just in case his doctor or someone else overlooked his genetic endowment while expecting him to gain average weight. Or if they were to express concern about him not maintaining the growth curves that represented his weight and length at birth.

Key times for catch-down growth are:

- Directly following birth. This is more common in the case of breast-fed babies, who have increased ability to self-regulate their milk intake from an earlier age compared to bottle-fed babies; and
- Around three months when a baby's sucking reflex has disappeared. At this time all healthy babies have a greater ability to self-regulate their intake to match growth needs

However, catch-down growth can occur at other times. After birth, Isabelle was placed on steroid medications to treat a medical condition. As a result her weight skyrocketed to above the 97th percentile, but her length remained consistent around the 25th percentile. Medications were ceased when she was five months of age and while she continued to growth length-wise, she gained very little weight over the next three months.

Once a baby can physically self-regulate her dietary intake, and provided parents allow her to do so by responding to her cues of hunger and fullness, her weight will head towards to her genetically determined course.

Average weekly weight gains and milk estimations based on age and weight will not apply to babies undergoing catch-down growth.

During the catch-down growth phase – which could last weeks or months – a baby may eat less and gain less than expected. Her weight, and in some cases length, will slowly drop to lower percentile curves on an infant growth chart until her size and shape realigns with her genetically determined path, at which time her growth then follows percentile curves that represent her natural body shape and size.

Catch-down growth is often mistaken as poor growth. The following table describes ways the two can differ.

Table 7.2: Catch-down growth versus poor growth

Catch-down growth	Poor growth
Natural decline in rate of growth.	**Abnormal** decline in rate of growth.
Growth heads **towards** genetically determined path.	Growth heads **away from** genetically determined path.
Baby **displays signs** of being well fed.	Baby **does not display** signs of being well fed.
Baby was born unusually large or has a **recent** history of excessive weight gain.	Baby could have a past history of excessive growth.

Constitutional growth delay

Constitutional growth delay (CGD) is another example of a **normal variation** of growth often mistaken as poor growth.

CGD involves a temporary delay in skeletal growth. Baby is usually normal size at birth. Starting from around three to six months of age her rate of growth is much slower than considered typical for a baby of her age and size. Weight gains are consistently below average. Tracking her growth on an infant growth chart shows a downward trend as her weight and length cross through multiple growth curves until two to three years of age. At that time, her growth resumes at a normal rate but her length remains below or parallel to the 3rd percentile until she reaches puberty. Her weight will be at a similar, but not necessarily the same, percentile curve. As a child she remains small in comparison to her peers and the heights of her parents until after puberty when her size returns to normal adult height relative to her parents' heights.

Usually, a parent or other close family member displayed a similar pattern of growth as a baby and child. They may have been called a 'late bloomer' who was smaller than most other children of the same age, but ultimately grew to adult height consistent with parents' heights. CGD can be distinguished from poor growth by x-raying a child's wrist. This shows delayed 'bone age', which means that her skeletal maturation is younger than her age in months or years.

This normal variation of growth can cause unnecessary anxiety for parents if it's not recognized. A CGD baby's appetite is less than expected because growth occurs at a slower rate compared to most babies her age.

When parents and health professionals overlook CGD, baby's lower than expected weight gain and the progressive pattern of weight and length dropping to lower percentile curves is usually mistaken as poor growth, which may then be wrongly blamed on insufficient food. This can result in a perfectly normal healthy baby being pressured to eat more than she needs.

In addition to these normal variations in infant growth, a number of false alarms can occur when weighing a baby that may make it appear as if she has gained poorly.

False alarms mistaken as poor growth

False alarms, though not variants in normal growth, are often mistaken as poor growth. Two common reasons for false alarms are fluctuations in bodily fluids and using different scales.

Fluctuations in bodily fluids

Bodily fluids, ie, baby's hydration level, volume of urine in her bladder, amount of food in her stomach and intestinal tract, fluctuate constantly over a 24-hour period. Fluctuations in bodily fluids can distort weight measurements from week to week. For example, last week baby might have been weighed **after** a feed. At the time, she also had a full bladder and might not have had a bowel motion for a day or two. This week, she's weighed **before** a feed. Just prior to heading out for her health check she had a large bowel motion and emptied her bladder. When she's weighed it **appears like** she has gained poorly or lost weight during the past week, when this might not be the case.

Fluctuations in bodily fluids can cause variations in weight of up to four ounces (113 grams) for a small baby and up to eight ounces (226 grams) for large babies when weighed at different times **on the same day.**

Weighing baby on different scales

Scales need to be regularly calibrated to ensure accuracy. If the same scales are used each time a baby is weighed then it doesn't matter if they're a little out of kilter. However, if baby is weighed on different scales, there could be a small or significant difference depending on whether each set of scales has been calibrated or not.

Mistake 4: Assuming baby is not eating enough

The most concerning of all mistakes when it **appears like** baby has gained poorly, because she didn't gain an expected amount, is that it's

automatically assumed to be because a nursing mother is not producing enough milk or a bottle-fed baby is not drinking enough. And as a result, the parent is **not** asked relevant questions about baby's nutritional state to check if this is the case or not. (See signs of well-fed baby in Chapter 6 for information needed before drawing conclusions.)

Asking the parent questions to identify if their baby's nutritional needs are met is an **essential** part of the assessment process, especially when it **appears like** a baby is drinking or gaining less than expected. This must be done in order to tell the difference between a genuine growth problem and a normal variation in infant growth or false alarm. And thus avoid making erroneous assumptions that can lead to poor feeding advice.

Make sure the assessment is correct

If you have been told that your baby's growth was poor when in reality she gained less than expected due to one of the reasons described in this chapter, you need to know. If your health professional has made a mistake he/she might not realize and could do the same again.

Your health professional won't be the one affected by a mistaken assessment of your baby's growth. Rather it could have negative consequences for your baby and family. Making a mistake about baby's growth, though causing you needless worry, is not the main concern. It's flawed feeding advice that follows, and the actions you might take as a result of **mistakenly believing** your baby's growth is poor that can cause infant feeding and growth problems.

If your baby is not gaining as expected, don't immediately jump to the conclusion that it is poor growth due to her not eating enough. Look for signs that indicate if your baby is well fed (see Chapter 6). If she displays such signs, she's eating enough and healthy growth will follow. In this case, have her weighed again a week later.

A single weight measurement is not as important as your baby's growth pattern over time. An infant growth chart provides a broader perspective of growth. Monitoring her growth **over time,** keeping in mind her inherited traits, provides a more accurate picture of her growth compared to the amount gained from one week to the next.

Some babies are more vulnerable to developing a feeding aversion compared to others, because their growth is not typical or their parents are more likely to receive poor feeding advice that results in baby being pressured to feed. To discover if this has been the case for your baby read on.

8

Babies at risk

Alex was born at 27 weeks. He was in hospital for three months. We were so excited when we finally took him home. He was feeding great for the first six weeks at home, but then started to get really upset while eating and not wanting to finish his bottles. In the past month it's gotten worse. He now screams as soon as we lay him in our arms to feed. His doctor said preterm babies are prone to feeding problems. He said if things don't get better soon he might need a feeding tube. I am so stressed. Do you think you can help? – Hannah

Alex's doctor is right. Preterm babies are prone to feeding problems, feeding aversion in particular, mainly due to one or more of the reasons we've already discussed: trying to control how much they take and unrealistic expectations about milk intake or growth. But it's not just preterm babies who are susceptible. Any baby who doesn't fit the 'average' or 'typical' mould in regards to growth is at increased risk because he's more likely to be pressured to feed compared to babies who follow a textbook pattern of growth.

This includes:

- preterm babies
- IUGR (intra-uterine growth restricted) babies
- short stature babies
- large at birth babies
- babies who underfeed in their early months
- babies who overfeed in their early months
- genetically lean babies and
- babies born to highly anxious parents.

This includes a lot of babies! From reading the previous chapters, you undoubtedly already appreciate why these babies could be at risk of developing a behavioral feeding aversion. However, there are circumstances unique to each group of babies that increase the likelihood of a behavioral feeding aversion.

While your baby may or may not fall into one these groups, I encourage you to read this chapter as the reasons these babies are vulnerable to developing a feeding aversion might apply to your baby.

Preterm babies

Many of the feeding strategies necessary to **support** a preterm baby to feed will at some point morph into **pressure** if parents keep trying to control how much their baby eats. Especially if they do this beyond the age when he can self-regulate his intake (decide when and how much he will eat).

If you're the parent of a preterm baby, whether you realize it or not, it's likely that you have been conditioned by health professionals to think 'numbers'. For example, the number of hours between feeds, the number of ounces or milliliters your baby must have each feed, and the number of ounces or grams your baby should gain each week. You may have been led to believe that you must control his feeds to make sure he drinks the recommended amount, which you may have needed to do for a brief period in his life ... but not forever.

In general, health professionals' focus is firmly fixed on ensuring preterm babies receive a specific volume of milk and that their growth is within an acceptable range, and not on a baby's enjoyment in feeding. And so parents of preterm babies are rarely told that they need to alter their infant feeding practices as baby matures; **from controlling** how much baby drinks **to supporting** baby to self-regulate his intake. Because they're unaware, they may continue to try to control the amount of milk their baby drinks for too long.

Attempting to control a baby's feeds beyond eight weeks adjusted age – which commonly occurs in the case of preterm babies – is why I believe preterm babies have a higher incidence of **feeding aversion** compared to term babies.

A serious error, which should not happen but does, is that some health professionals continue to calculate babies' milk requirements at the preterm rate for longer than they should. More often, overestimation occurs due to an oversight. Parents need to use different calculations when estimating their baby's milk requirements as he matures, but many are not informed. As a result, they might use pressure tactics to make their baby drink an amount of milk that in some cases is a gross overestimation.

IUGR (intra-uterine growth restricted) babies

There are two types of IUGR: **Asymmetrical IUGR** meaning when baby is born he's of normal length considering his parents' heights, but he looks skinny or malnourished; and **symmetrical IUGR** where a baby is born unusually tiny for his gestational age, and much shorter than expected considering his parents' heights, but he has a healthy layer of body fat.

An IUGR baby might not be given the chance to decide how much his body needs. It's commonly assumed that because he's underweight or smaller than expected – which is due to circumstances in the womb beyond baby's control, such as placental insufficiency – that he's incapable of deciding what his body needs after birth. But provided baby is physically and neurologically healthy, this is not the case.

> The doctor said Oliver needs at least a minimum of 24 ounces (680 ml) a day. Each feed can take over an hour but I try to make sure he gets this because I am always paranoid that he won't gain enough weight. Everyone wants a chubby baby, right, because they think they are 'healthy'. At night he drinks just fine and can drink the whole bottle in 15 minutes. I don't understand why he seems to hate feeding in the day. – Laura

While it is important that Oliver gets enough to eat, he's not getting the chance to decide what this amount is. Laura decides what's 'enough' based on her doctor's recommendations, and she tries to make Oliver drink this amount whether he wants it, or needs it, or not.

Oliver is at serious risk of developing an aversion to feeding if Laura doesn't let him decide how much to drink.

Everyone wants to see a baby gaining weight, especially in the case of an IUGR baby. It's believed to be safer to offer a baby a little more milk than he might need than not offer enough. So health professionals have a tendency to overestimate milk volumes required to enable catch-up growth. There's no harm in offering a baby more than he might need. However, if parents pressure or force their baby to drink a 'must have' amount, this could cause him to become averse to feeding.

TRUE OR FALSE?

1. Rapid weight gain is good.

TRUE & FALSE: Rapid weight gain can be healthy if it's achieved at baby's pace. In other words, he's allowed to decide how much food his body needs. But if rapid growth is thrust upon a baby as a result of force-feeding or tube feeding, this is not necessarily healthy. Forcing a baby to drink more than he wants can override his inborn ability to self-regulate his intake, teaches him to overeat, and thus increase the risk of obesity problems in the future.

2. More food equals faster growth.

TRUE & FALSE: If a baby is born underweight, as is the case of a skinny asymmetrical IUGR baby, or he becomes underweight due to underfeeding, more food might improve growth provided lack of nutrition is the cause. However, if a baby already has a healthy layer of body fat, as can be the case for symmetrical IUGR babies and genetically short statured babies born to small parents, more food might increase body fat, but it will not increase the rate of baby's skeletal growth. In other words his length won't climb

---

to higher percentiles on an infant growth chart any faster than it would have if he were allowed to decide how much to eat.

It's not hard to overfeed a baby while his sucking reflex is present. In some cases overfeeding can cause poor growth. An overfed baby may vomit, but he won't necessarily vomit up only the excess. Once vomiting mechanisms are triggered, he might vomit the entire contents of his stomach. In some cases less can be more; less food, less vomiting, better growth. (See overfeeding in Chapter 5.)

Short stature babies

Short stature babies include familial (genetic or inherited) short babies born to short parents and symmetrical IUGR babies.

An unrealistic expectation about growth may result in a short statured baby being pressured to feed. This can occur because some health professionals erroneously consider average weekly weight gain figures as 'pass or fail' measurements. Or due to an expectation that a baby's weight and length 'should' climb to higher growth curves.

A baby born to short parents will not regularly gain average weight because he's not genetically inclined to be of average size. He may gain less than average and follow lower percentile curves on an infant growth chart.

A symmetrical IUGR baby might be small or petite and yet be born to parents who are average height or taller. So while he's not inherently predisposed to be small, he may gain less than average and his weight and length remain on lower percentile curves. Some symmetrically IUGR babies will catch up to the size expected according to inherited traits, and their weight and length climb to higher percentile curves, but this can take up to two years to do so. Not all IUGR babies will catch up completely. Some will remain small.

Large at birth babies

Some babies are born large, but are not genetically inclined to be so. They may have laid down extra stores of body fat in the womb for various reasons, such as maternal diabetes, maternal diet, and certain medications.

Or they were born proportionate but unexpectedly large in relation to their parents' heights. These babies may go through a period of catch-down growth in the early months as their bodies realign to their genetically determined growth path. When baby gains less than expected, this may be mistaken as poor growth assumed to be because baby is either not receiving or not eating enough. But this isn't correct. (See Chapter 7 for more on catch-down growth.)

Noah's case provides and example of just how bad things can get when catch-down growth is mistaken as poor growth.

Baby Noah

Noah was born weighing 9 pounds (lb) 12 ounces (oz) or 4.42 kilograms (kg). This placed his weight above the 97th percentile on an infant growth chart. His length was 19 inches (48.25 cm), which meant his length was around the 25th percentile. His mother Michelle was 5'3" (160 cm) and father Brett 5'8" (173 cm). So Noah's length was in keeping with his genetic endowment, but his weight was a surprise to his family.

Noah was exclusively breast-fed from birth. His weight at three weeks of age indicated he was 3.5 oz (100 g) above his birth weight, which is well below average. The health nurse told Michelle that she had low milk supply and advised her to supplement Noah's breastfeeds with infant formula. This created doubts in Michelle's mind about her ability to successfully breastfeed and by the time Noah was five-weeks-old he was completely formula-fed.

Noah initially fed well from a bottle and gained close to average weight each week. However, the situation changed around the age of two months. He started to drink less than the recommended amount of formula based on his age and weight, and his weight gain slowed. Michelle found she needed to use pressure to try to get Noah to drink the recommended amount, but never quite succeeded.

By three months of age his weight was around the 60th percentile. Noah would become quite distressed at feeding times. He would cry as soon as Michelle held him in a feeding position, buck and scream and turn his head into Michelle's chest, and try to bat the bottle away.

The child health nurse suspected acid reflux and advised Michelle to have Noah medically assessed. Her GP prescribed Ranitidine (an acid suppressing medication). But this didn't help. Noah was then referred to a pediatrician who prescribed Omeprazole (an even stronger acid suppressing medication) and Neocate (a hypoallergenic formula). Despite these treatments, there was no improvement in his feeding behavior.

At four months of age Noah's weight was around the 25th percentile. His milk intake dropped to between 13 to 16 oz (385 to 475 ml) a day. He was referred to a speech and language pathologist (SLP) who confirmed he had no underlying sucking problem. And also referred to a pediatric dietician who recommended increasing the calories he received by switching him to high-energy formula. But this resulted in him drinking even less. His pediatrician suggested that Michelle start feeding him solids. Noah initially enjoyed eating solids but within four weeks he was refusing to eat.

By six months his weight had dropped to the 7th percentile. His length stayed steady around the 25th. He was diagnosed as 'failure to thrive', referred to a pediatric gastroenterologist who admitted him to hospital for a series of diagnostic tests; all of which returned negative results. Out of options, his doctor recommended he be tube-fed. Michelle and Brett reluctantly agreed. Noah remained in hospital for 10 days, during which time he gained over 10 oz (300 g).

When Noah was eight months old, Michelle consulted

me about the possibility of tube weaning. Noah's growth was on track but he continued to reject bottle feeds and solids, and the situation didn't look like improving any time soon.

After taking a detailed history from Michelle, examining Noah's growth charts, and the feeding app that Michelle had used to keep records of feeds and wet diapers since birth, I suspected that Noah's catch-down growth had been overlooked. At birth he was 2.5 lb (more than a kilogram) heavier than the average sized baby, and yet he was shorter than average. I didn't need to see him to know that he carried generous rolls of fat on his body. Noah might have been born a chubby baby, but this didn't mean he was destined to remain that way. It would not be healthy if he did. He would be expected to go through a period of catch-down growth as his weight realigned with his genetically inherited body shape. His body started this process from birth but the process was halted temporarily when he was switched to bottle-feeding, which meant he could be pressured to drink for a time (until his sucking reflex disappeared and he was strong enough to resist).

Despite having gained less than average weight in the early weeks, according to the details recorded on Michelle's app, all signs pointed to Noah being a well-fed baby. There was nothing wrong with Michelle's milk supply at that time. What had been mistaken as poor growth due to low milk supply was catch-down growth. The consequence of the health nurse's mistaken assessment of Noah's growth and Michelle's milk supply – which was assumed to be low without feeding observation or any other form of assessment – was feeding recommendations that led to Michelle ceasing breastfeeding long before she had planned to. (Michelle's loss in confidence in her ability to breastfeed could also have a negative impact on any future babies she might have.) But this was not the only time Michelle and Noah were let down.

Once Noah was fully formula-fed, the nurse then overestimated his formula requirements. She used standard calculations based on age and weight, but did not take into account the fact that Noah was still carrying excess stores of body fat, or that his requirements might be less and weight gains lower because he would be expected to go through a period of catch-down growth. Noah should have been allowed to take the amount he wanted according to his hunger and satiety cues, which reflected his growth needs, but he was not.

Thinking she was doing the right thing, Michelle forced him to take an overly inflated volume of milk until she could no longer do so when Noah was three months of age. By force-feeding, Michelle had caused Noah to develop a feeding aversion. As a result of his aversion his milk volumes dropped below his needs. He burned up fat reserves at a rapid rate until there was little left. What had initially been mistaken as poor growth became poor growth.

Michelle and Brett did everything they could to find answers to why Noah hated eating. The health nurse, GP, pediatrician, GI specialist, SLP and dietician all assumed his fierce rejection of feeding and poor growth was to due to acid reflux and milk protein allergy. Had his aversive feeding behavior been due to these reasons, acid reflux medications and hypoallergenic formula would have fixed the problem. According to Michelle none of the many health professionals she consulted asked about her feeding practices, or observed her feeding Noah. None considered the possibility of a behavioral feeding aversion due to being repeatedly pressured to feed from a bottle. And later pressured to eat solid foods which was the reason he became averse to eating solids after four weeks.

Noah had no underlying physical cause preventing him from feeding orally, so over a period of three weeks, he successfully weaned from tube feeds onto oral feeds once his aversion to bottle-feeding was no longer reinforced. After weaning to bottle-feeds, which he enjoyed now he was no longer pressured to eat, he went on to relish eating solids as well, which were also offered without pressure. Noah was weaned off acid suppressing medications and returned to regular infant formula without ill effects. Michelle allowed him to decide how much he would eat and Noah continued to gain weight well. After eight long months, Michelle and Brett were finally free to enjoy life with Noah without the stress of constantly trying to make him eat. And Michelle would be better prepared in the future if she were to give birth to another large baby.

I wish I could say that Noah's case was exceptional, but it's not. I see similar scenarios in many bottle-feeding aversion cases. But most don't get to the point of being tube-fed.

When errors, oversights and mistaken assumptions made by health professionals trigger the sequence of events that leads to babies developing feeding aversions, it's families that pay. For families like Noah's, it can be a hefty toll. Michelle was diagnosed with post-partum depression when Noah was five months old. Maybe this would have occurred even if she hadn't endured unrelenting stress for months because of Noah's feeding issues. But she will never know.

Babies who underfeed in their early months

A baby could be born a healthy weight in relation to his length and after birth gain weight very slowly due to underfeeding.

Unfortunately, health professionals in general don't allocate sufficient time to thoroughly assess a baby's growth and identify and address common reasons for poor growth, such as breastfeeding latch problems, rigid feeding schedules, unsuitable or faulty feeding equipment or infant sleep deprivation. Instead it's assumed that baby's poor growth is because a breastfeeding mother has insufficient milk supply, or the parent is not offering their bottle-fed baby enough milk, or the parent is not fulfilling their responsibility to 'make sure' baby drinks the recommended amount. (Note: Parents are **not** responsible for baby drinking a predetermined amount – see Chapter 5 for parents' infant feeding responsibilities.) As a result, breastfeeding mothers are advised to supplement breastfeeds with infant formula and parents of bottle-fed babies are told to make sure their baby eats a specified minimum amount each feed.

Out of concern for baby's health, a parent will reluctantly resort to pressure or force to get a lean or underweight baby to feed, because they know no other way to get him to consume enough milk for healthy growth. By pressuring baby this can cause a feeding aversion, which then turns baby off feeding, compounding the problem originally causing underfeeding.

Babies who overfeed in their early months

> Jack has been bottle-fed since birth. He has always been a great feeder, until now. I used to feed him every three hours and he would finish his bottle every time. Now (aged 2 months) he has started to leave a lot of milk in the bottle. If I try to make him finish, he screams. Why does he suddenly not want to eat? – Caroline

Jack is now at an age where he can decide how much he wants to drink. I can 'see' by his weight and length measurements that he's a chubby baby. I check his growth pattern since birth. His weight gains up until last week have been huge. It's likely that he has been overfeeding or overfed since birth. The fact that he has accumulated generous rolls of body fat in recent months, plus his newfound ability to self-regulate his milk intake, means he now drinks less than estimated using standard calculations based on age and weight.

I suspect Jack is screaming when Caroline 'tries to make him finish' because Caroline is not responding according to his satiety cues and stopping the feed. Caroline needs to allow Jack to decide what his body needs. If she doesn't, she could be setting him up for a feeding aversion. Caroline also needs to realize that Jack may drink and gain less than average based on his age and weight, as his body shape readjusts according to his genetic endowment.

An overfed baby is not necessarily a chubby baby. (See Chapter 5 for reasons.) Even tiny preterm babies and skinny IUGR babies can overfeed. When a previously overfed baby's milk intake drops and/or weight gain slows most people find this confusing. They assume that baby should be drinking more now that he's bigger. Alarmed, the parent loses trust that baby will take what he needs, and starts to ignore behavioral cues that indicate he's no longer hungry, and persist in trying to make him consume the amount he was taking previously. By ignoring baby's satiety cues and pressuring him to feed, this increases the chances that he will develop an aversion to feeding.

Genetically lean babies

You can't fight your genes. Your body shape is programmed into your DNA. As adults, we might accumulate excess body fat because we eat for the wrong reasons, such as when we're bored, tired, as a reward, when anxious or upset and so on. Babies, unlike adults, eat for the right reason – hunger.

A baby who is averse to feeding will try to ignore his hunger cues, but he will eat according to hunger when he learns to enjoy feeding once again. Once a baby is over his feeding aversion and allowed to decide when and how much he will eat, his body shape and size will follow his genetically determined path. Some babies are naturally inclined to be chubbier and some leaner than others.

As a society we think that chubby babies are healthy babies and that lean babies are underfed. No one is concerned when baby is chubby, but everyone makes comment if a baby is lean. Babies don't need to be average or above average weight or carry generous layers of body fat in order to be healthy. When a baby is lean the reason should be investigated, but a percentage of babies, like Aiden, are genetically inclined to be lean.

Baby Aiden

Aiden was born average weight and length. But starting from around eight weeks of age, the amount of milk he drank was less than expected and his weekly weight gains were lower than average. Aiden's mother, Evelyn, would spend most of her day and night trying to make him eat the recommended amount. Each feed Aiden was pressured for over an hour. What he did not drink while awake, Evelyn would try to make him take while sleeping. Evelyn stated her entire day revolved around trying to make sure Aiden got enough to eat. But as much as she tried she could not get him to eat the recommended amount.

By three months of age Aiden was classified as 'failure to thrive'. As the weeks passed all the usual reflux medications and formula changes were tried without improvement in his feeding or growth, and the decision was made to tube-feed him. The plan was to let him eat what he wanted to eat but then top him up to a specified amount of formula through the tube. Within less than a week he stopped feeding orally and was totally tube-fed. He vomited after every feed. Evelyn felt she could not move him or play with him for fear he would vomit. He was switched to high-energy formula to provide more calories in a lower volume and given prokinetic medications to speed up gastric emptying time, but still he vomited. He was often gassy and uncomfortable and slept poorly. But he did gain some weight, and his weight slowly edged into the lower end of what is generally considered as a normal range in relation to his length.

At six months of age Aiden's parents consulted with me about weaning him from tube feeds to bottle-feeding. I suspected he was averse to bottle-feeding due to being forced-fed in the past and currently being 'encouraged' (unsuccessfully) to take a bottle using gentler forms of pressure. So this needed to be addressed. I recommended they switch him back to normal strength formula. He was successfully weaned over two weeks. After tube weaning Aiden would get excited at the sight of the bottle when he was hungry, grab it, bring it to his own mouth, feed contently, and stop sucking in a relaxed state when he was done. But he only ate about three-quarters of the calories his parents had been told he needed. Worried, they were advised by the dietician to give him high-energy milk once again, but this resulted in a drop in the amount he would eat. He received roughly the same number of calories either way. Proving to be of no benefit, they returned him to regular strength formula so that he would receive more fluids.

Over the next month Aiden gained very little and his body mass index (which provides a rough estimation of body fat) dropped below the range considered as normal, placing him back into the underweight category.

His parents were understandably worried. Yet despite not drinking or gaining as much as expected Aiden was far happier now that he was deciding how much he would drink. He seldom vomited, was no longer gassy, slept better, he was more energetic, he was laughing for the first time, and interacted with his parents and others more than he did while being tube-fed. He also developed a few new skills, rolling and then sitting, in rapid succession (as a result of no longer needing to be restrained to prevent him from pulling out the tube), and from being able to placed on a blanket on the floor to play without the fear of him vomiting up his feed.

Even though Aiden's body mass index indicated he was in the underweight category, he had fat on his body, just not as much as he had previously when tube-fed or as much as the 'average' baby has. Apart from being lean, Aiden displayed all the signs that he was well fed (see Chapter 6).

Both his parents were lean, his dad, Marcus, in particular. I asked about other family members. Marcus' parents and siblings were all very lean. Interestingly, Marcus had been diagnosed as 'failure to thrive' as a baby, he remained lean as a child and was now lean as an adult. Apparently, he has been considered to be underweight all of his life.

I suspected that Aiden was also genetically inclined to be lean. Over the next few months his weight continued to follow a growth curve three percentiles below his length, medically classified as underweight, but he remained a happy energetic baby who was into everything, and it became clear that he is naturally inclined to be leaner than most other babies.

If your baby is genetically inclined to be lean, you're not going to fatten him up by making him eat more than he's willing to eat. Even if you do manage to make him to eat more by force or a feeding tube, his homeostatic mechanisms will probably kick in to regulate his intake according to his needs. He might throw up and pass more frequent or extra large stools and still not gain extra body fat. (See overfeeding in Chapter 5.)

You can't change your baby's natural body shape, but you can change your expectations.

Babies with highly anxious parents

> The doc says Sebastian (aged 5 months) will eat what he needs and we can see how that goes when we weigh him. But the internet says he should be eating at least 2 oz for every pound, so 28 oz, and I see most babies at our moms group eating upwards of 30 oz at his age. I can only get him to take 22–26 oz. – Jane

Jane received great advice from her doctor, but she wanted a target figure to aim for to feel confident that Sebastian was getting enough. While 2 oz/lb/day (120 ml/kg/day) is average for a baby of Sebastian's age, it may be more than he needs. Or he could be taking less than he needs due to a feeding aversion. After further questioning, Jane acknowledged that she was using pressure to try to make him eat 28 oz a day. Jane will not know how much Sebastian needs for healthy growth until he gets over his aversion and is allowed to decide how much his body needs.

Some parents – by their own admission – confess to having a strong desire to 'control' any given situation. Others may have been traumatized by experiences related to this baby's or a previous baby's feeding, like baby being admitted to hospital due to refusing to eat. So the desire to control baby's feeds stems from an overwhelming need to avoid a similar stressful situation. For whatever reason, a parent may have a set figure in mind that baby 'must' drink and as a result overlook or disregard baby's satiety cues and use pressure to control how much he eats. And in doing so they make the feeding experience unpleasant or stressful for their baby, which when repeated, cause him to become averse to feeding.

Other babies at risk of feeding aversion

Other babies who might be pressured to feed include:
- babies who are very sleepy following birth due to jaundice or other reasons
- babies who experienced hypoglycemia following birth

- babies weaned from the breast who may be taking time to get the hang of sucking from a bottle. (Drinking from a bottle is a learned skill once baby's sucking reflex has disappeared.)
- babies recovering from surgery who are not gaining weight quickly enough for their health professional's liking
- constitutional growth delay babies
- babies with syndromes or metabolic disorders that affect their growth
- tube-fed babies whose parents are trying to get to bottle-feed.

A feeding aversion is not exclusive to the babies listed in this chapter. However, this chapter demonstrates a number of scenarios that might cause parents to believe, or be advised by their health professional, that they must take charge over their baby's feeding to make sure he drinks 'enough'.

By this point, you have now discovered the cause of your baby's feeding aversion and possibly the reason this situation developed. It's now time to learn how to encourage your baby to enjoy feeding once again.

PART C: Solutions

9

Five Steps to Success

> Your feeding recommendations worked. I am so happy. Erin used to scream when I tried to give her a bottle but now she gets excited when she sees it. She holds onto it herself and happily drinks the whole bottle in one go. She even feeds when we are out, so we can finally leave the house and enjoy doing normal family things. We can't thank you enough. You have changed our lives.
> – Tegan

I am delighted to learn that Erin now enjoys feeding. This is a stark contrast to how she fed two weeks ago. She previously did everything she could to try to avoid feeding. The removal of the constant stress caused from worrying if your precious baby will eat enough to thrive is life changing for families. Now both Erin and Tegan can enjoy this special time together.

Feeding times should be enjoyable for baby and parents. While this might not be the case right now, it can be. To encourage your baby to go from loathing to loving feeding, I recommend the following steps:

---

5 STEPS TO SUCCESS

Step 1: Ensure baby is healthy.
Step 2: Plan to succeed.
Step 3: Motivate baby to feed.
Step 4: Follow baby's lead.
Step 5: Support baby's sleep.

I will explain what each step involves.

Step 1: Ensure baby is healthy

Before considering a change in your current infant feeding management, it's essential that your baby be in good health.

Baby needs to be physically well. Any illness could decrease her appetite and the chances of successfully resolving her feeding aversion. If you're unsure about her state of health, have her examined by a doctor.

Baby has to be capable of feeding safely from a bottle. Please consult your baby's doctor or have her checked by a speech and language pathologist (SLP) if you have doubts.

Baby ideally has a healthy layer of body fat. Most babies will lose a little weight during the early days when parents follow my feeding recommendations, but return to their starting weight within one to two weeks. Based on my experience a loss of between 2 to 10 ounces (60 to 300 grams) is typical. Lean babies tend to lose less than chubby babies, probably because they have less to lose. However, it's not possible to predict exactly how much weight a baby might lose or how long it could take her to regain this weight.

What if baby is underweight? It's not unusual for a baby who is averse to feeding to be underweight. If your baby is underweight, you can still follow my **Five Steps to Success**. However, I recommend that you have your baby examined by a doctor to check for any underlying physical problems that might be contributing to poor growth, which may require treatment. This is usually one of the first things parents do, so you have probably already done so. Also, ask baby's doctor or health nurse if he or she will help you monitor her weight and progress during the process of resolving her feeding aversion.

Continue medications

Though you'll be continuing all prescribed medications, don't add them to your baby's bottle. Many medications have a bitter taste, which might turn her off feeding.

Avoid giving medications directly before bottle-feeds. Trying to feed her when she's already upset because you made her take nasty tasting meds is not ideal when you want her to enjoy bottle-feeding.

If medications were prescribed to treat your baby's feeding aversion, and her aversion is resolved as a result of following the strategies in this book, ask her doctor whether she needs medications. It's typically assumed that a baby's aversive feeding behavior occurs as a result of a medical condition such as acid reflux, but it's seldom the case. But wait until she's over her feeding aversion.

Continue milk additives or high-energy feeds

Continue milk additives or high-energy feeds as you have been advised. However, take into account that the extra calories will mean your baby drinks lower volumes. Once she's over her feeding aversion, consider getting her back to regular strength formula or breast milk, which will provide more fluids for the same number of calories. This can be done gradually under the guidance of your healthcare professional.

Step 2: Plan to succeed

Think about ways to reduce yours and your baby's stress levels.

Prioritize

Prioritize fixing your baby's feeding aversion for a two-week period. Skip or delay anything that is not essential that might upset her during that time. Any upset could cause a minor or major setback. Where possible reduce your workload and responsibilities during this time so that your focus can remain on resolving your baby's feeding issues once and for all.

Plan for baby to be at home

Plan for your baby to be at home for all feeds during this process. You have no doubt already discovered that she doesn't feed well while out. This is because an unfamiliar environment is stimulating. It could mean she's too interested in looking around to eat. Or she becomes too upset by the extra stimulation of a new environment to feed at a time when she's hungry and still apprehensive about feeding.

(Her apprehension will not be because of my feeding recommendations, rather her memory of being pressured to feed.)

If it's simply not possible to feed her at home for each feed, then aim to be at home as much as possible. Once she's no longer averse to bottle-feeding you may find she will be happy to feed wherever she happens to be at the time.

Limit the number of people feeding baby

Ideally, one of baby's main caregivers, mom or dad, will provide all feeds throughout this process. If it's not possible for one person, then try to limit the number to two. The more people feeding baby, the longer the process can take and the greater the risk that someone will unintentionally and unknowingly pressure her, reducing the chance of successfully resolving her feeding aversion.

Once your baby is over her feeding aversion, it will be okay for others to feed her. But it's essential that you inform them that they **must not** pressure her to eat more than she's willing to eat. Any pressure could cause her to relapse. You may need to describe subtle forms of pressure (see Chapter 3) as they might mistakenly consider these as encouragement or helping baby to feed.

Get support

This might be physical support, perhaps to take care of other children, cook or do housework while you focus on resolving baby's feeding issues. Or emotional support to help you avoid lapsing into old habits, such as trying to pressure her to feed. Your partner, a family member, friend or health professional may be able to provide support.

A health professional, such as baby's doctor or health nurse might also be able to support you to monitor her progress. If you're not receiving professional support, but feel it would be helpful, book a consultation with a health professional experienced in resolving infant feeding aversions through my website **www.babycareadvice.com**.

Step 3: Motivate baby to feed

There's nothing more effective than a hungry little tummy to motivate a baby to feed. However, a baby who has become apprehensive or fearful of feeding will go beyond the level of hunger sufficient to motivate a baby **who is not averse to feeding** to want eat, before she will willingly eat.

Without hunger there will be no incentive for your baby to want to eat. To help motivate her you need to:

- cease sleep-feeding (bottle-feeding baby in a drowsy state or while sleeping)
- temporarily stop giving her solids and/or breastfeeding her during the day and
- stop giving her milk by any means other than a bottle, such as a syringe, spoon or sippy cup.

If your baby's daily milk intake is very low there may be exceptions (these are described in Chapter 10). Wait until your baby is over her bottle-feeding aversion before recommencing solids or returning to breastfeeding her during the day.

Note: If you temporarily cease breastfeeding during the day to encourage her acceptance of bottle-feeds, there is the possibility that she could start to prefer bottle-feeds and reject breastfeeds. (This risk occurs with any baby who is both breast- and bottle-fed.) Only you can decide whether getting her to willingly feed from a bottle is worth this risk.

A hungry tummy is a great motivator! However, when a baby is averse to feeding, hunger alone won't encourage her to eat enough for healthy growth. While she's wary about being pressured – which she will continue to be for some time after you have removed pressure – she will take only small amounts, just enough to soothe the pangs of hunger, before stopping. Before she will eat to satisfaction, your baby needs to learn that feeding is enjoyable. Step 4 explains how you make the experience enjoyable.

Step 4: Follow your baby's lead

A baby's behavior is a reflection of her intentions and feelings. She avoids the bottle or displays conflicted feeding behavior when her previous feeding experiences have been unpleasant or stressful. To make the experience pleasurable, you need to remove **all** pressure to feed, both subtle and obvious.

Don't expect your baby to suddenly go from avoidance to delight in feeding because you stop trying to make her eat. Removing pressure is essential, but it's only part of the process. You need to regain your baby's trust before she will get over her aversion. You can achieve this by demonstrating that **you trust your baby** to decide when and how much to eat

– even though you might not feel you can at present – by responding appropriately and quickly to her cues when she shows interest in feeding and disinterest or rejection of feeds. (How to respond is described in Chapter 10.)

> **Trust in a child's inborn ability to regulate his/her dietary intake is the key to preventing and solving many infant and childhood feeding problems.**

Only once your baby is over her fear of feeding and allowed to self-regulate her dietary intake can she show you she's worthy of your trust by eating enough for healthy growth. But she can only show you if you have enough trust in her to let her reach that point.

Step 5: Support baby's sleep

Feeding and sleeping are closely linked. If your baby doesn't feed well she might not sleep well. Equally, if she doesn't sleep well she might not feed well. Ensuring a baby receives adequate sleep can be challenging at the best of times. It's going to be harder if she's hungry, which is likely in the early stages of resolving her aversion. Chapter 12 describes ways to support your baby's sleep throughout this process.

How long will it take?

It's a slow process to undo a baby's negative feelings about feeding and replace these with positive ones. She needs **repeated** positive feeding experiences where her cues are responded to **before** she will feel its safe to eat, **before** she gains confidence that she's no longer going to be pressured to eat, and **before** she will relax, enjoy feeding and continue to contentedly suck until satisfied. This doesn't happen overnight. Based on my experience, two weeks is the average timeframe involved in resolving a baby's aversion to bottle-feeding. But this can range from one to four weeks.

Next I describe how to manage your baby's feeds to promote enjoyment.

10
Feeding management

> Thank you for explaining what Aaron's behavior means and how to respond. No one has ever told me this before. I didn't realize that as he got older I needed to get his permission before putting the nipple into his mouth. Now I see that I previously mistook his screaming as pain when it was him shouting at me to stop trying to make him eat. I only wish I had known this sooner. I feel so bad that I have caused him to hate feeding.
> – Shelly

Aaron is now three months old. When he was born Shelly was taught **parent-directed** feeding methods – where the parent decides and controls when and how much baby eats, and baby is expected to comply. However, she needed to switch to **baby-led** feeding practices – where baby is allowed to choose when and how much he will eat, and the parent responds accordingly – once Aaron was old enough to signal hunger and fullness. Ideally, Shelly should have adjusted her feeding practices at least a month ago, possibly sooner, but no one advised her to do so. And so she continued to try to control Aaron's feeds. This resulted in a battle of wills that led to him rejecting feeds.

When a baby has become averse to feeding, it's seldom sufficient to simplistically advise parents to stop pressuring their baby feed. What 'pressure' means is open to interpretation. So I provide parents with a list of feeding rules and recommendations that are highly effective in reversing a baby's negative feelings about bottle-feeding. These are explained in this and the following three chapters. You will also find a checklist of rules and recommendations in Chapter 14.

We begin with the golden rules.

Golden feeding rules

There are four feeding rules I call golden rules because they must be followed in order to reverse a baby's negative feelings about feeding. These are:

GOLDEN FEEDING RULES

1. No pressure to feed.
2. No sleep-feeding.
3. Bottle-feeds only.
4. Follow baby's lead.

There are exceptions to these rules, which I will explain.

Rule 1: No pressure to feed

If the stress associated with being pressured to feed is the reason your baby would rather go hungry than eat, then continuing this pressure will reinforce his aversion. All pressure must end, including tactics that involve coercion, cajoling, and trickery. (See Chapter 3 for examples.)

This means you must not pressure or 'encourage' baby to accept the bottle against his will, nor to drink more than he's willing to drink.

There are no exceptions to the 'No pressure' rule. This rule applies equally to day and night feeds.

'Day' and 'night' definitions

By 'day' I am referring to a 12-hour period, for example six am to six pm, or any other 12-hour period that best resembles your baby's day. 'Night' refers the remaining 12 hours.

Rule 2: No sleep-feeding

This means no feeding baby in a drowsy state or while sleeping **during the day.** You might have to compromise on this rule at night if your baby refuses to feed or takes very little during the day, which is possible in the early days involved in resolving his feeding aversion.

The reason for the exception - at night only - is to ensure adequate hydration so that he's not physically compromised, and also to support his sleep.

Rule 3: Bottle-feeds only

The more calories your baby receives by other methods, for example, solids, milk via syringe or sippy cup, or breastfeeding, the less incentive he will have to willingly accept bottle-feeds. There will be a point where he will get by on the calories provided in these ways and continue to reject bottle-feeds.

There are exceptions to provide milk using these methods at night if baby's milk intake during the day is low. You might also need to keep breastfeeding during the night to maintain his desire to breastfeed while resolving his aversion to bottle-feeding. However, this process will be less complicated if you stop giving baby solid foods until after his bottle-feeding aversion is resolved.

Rule 4: Follow baby's lead

This means respecting your baby's right to decide when he eats and how much he will eat. This is linked to the 'no pressure' rule but extends to being flexible about feeding times – not trying to stick to a feeding schedule – and providing a quick and appropriate response to his behavioral cues while feeding.

There are a few exceptions to the 'follow baby's lead' rule. As you read this chapter and the remaining chapters of this book, you will find situations where you might need to take the lead, not just with regards to his feeding but possibly sleeping as well. These will be explained.

Now the rules have been covered, next I will describe my feeding recommendations.

When to offer feeds

'Offer' means precisely that. Please don't mistake this with how often your baby 'should' feed. Your job is to offer. It's your baby's job to decide whether he will accept or reject your offer. He won't necessarily accept a feed each time you offer, especially in the early days.

While cue-based feeding (also called demand feeding) makes sense in theory, in practical terms it doesn't work well for every baby, for example:

- A baby who is averse to feeding could be fussing or crying due to hunger and reject your offer to feed him, and continue to fuss or cry. So if you were offering feeds based on hunger cues, this would mean you would be offering repeatedly; something I don't recommend you do because it can become harassment.
- Babies often fuss, cry, suck fists etc for reasons other than hunger and these can be easily mistaken as hunger. So cue-based feeding may mean you could be offering your baby feeds for the wrong reasons, and puzzled as to why he's rejecting. If he's expecting to be pressured, as he has been in the past, he might not react well to being offered a bottle when he's not hungry.
- Some babies have easy-going temperaments. They're non-demanding by nature. Cue-based feeding may mean baby goes too long before being offered a feed.

A **time-based feeding schedule** will also **not** work while resolving a baby's feeding aversion because at times he'll reject feeds or take very little. If he's upset due to hunger, it's not reasonable to make him wait until the clock indicates it's time for the next feed. He could become too distraught to feed if he's kept waiting too long.

If your baby is a twin (or other multiple-birth baby), it's understandable that you would want both babies feeding at the same time. This may be possible **after** he's over his feeding aversion and willingly eating well, but it's unlikely to be achievable **during** the process of resolving his aversion.

So when to offer baby feeds? It needs to be a **semi-demand pattern** – a balance between cue-based and time-based feeding – suitable for your baby. There is no set timeframe while resolving baby's aversion, as the balancing point will vary from feed to feed depending on his mood and how much he takes. Here are some tips on how to achieve a balance.

The first feed of the day

The 'first feed' occurs once your baby has woken for the day. Don't assume he's ready to eat just because his eyes have opened. Many of us are not ready to eat when we first wake. This is due to the lingering effect of appetite suppressing hormones released at night.

Give baby a chance to show he's hungry. Offer him a bottle-feed when he shows signs that might indicate hunger, such as fussing or sucking on fists or fingers.

Because some babies are non-demanding, you might need to offer him a feed 30 minutes after waking if he hasn't shown hunger cues before that time. But if you find he's more receptive to feeding if you wait longer, then do so.

Consecutive daytime feeds

How long to wait before offering the next feed would depend partially on your baby's behavior and partially on the clock. The recommendations below apply regardless of how much your baby took at the last feed or whether he completely rejected the last feed.

If baby's not fussing

If your baby is not showing signs of discomfort that could be attributed to hunger, then offer the next feed at around three hours. If he's napping at the time, don't wake him. Leave him to sleep. When he wakes, give him 15 minutes or so to see if he demands a feed, and if not offer one.

If your baby rejected the previous feed or took very little – to be expected in the early days – this will understandably cause you a great deal of anxiety. Try to avoid offering him a bottle-feed simply because you think 'He should be hungry by now.'

If baby is fussing

As already mentioned, a baby who is averse to feeding could be hungry and yet reject your offer or he might take only a little. In which case, it may not be long before he's fussing again due to hunger. If he has only just rejected your offer to feed him, there's a good chance he's going to reject again if you offer too soon. None of us like to be offered food repeatedly when we have said 'no'. The hungrier your baby becomes the more likely he will accept a feed. So you may need to soothe him as best you can and allow his hunger to build a little more.

It's possible that he could be fussing for reasons unrelated to hunger. So try a few delay tactics to soothe him as you wait for his hunger to build, such as playing, bathing, taking him for a walk in the stroller or carrier, or napping.

Only attempt to extend the time between feeds **while it's reasonable** to do so. If delay tactics are not soothing him, by all means offer him a feed, even if it's only been an hour since you last offered.

Don't become too fixated about when to offer. The most important thing is that you respect his right to decline your offer. And you avoid harassing him by repeated offers.

During the night

How to manage night feeds will vary according to your baby's age, milk intake during the day and whether he wakes or not.

When a baby is averse to feeding, he doesn't find feeding pleasurable and so he's going to try to avoid feeding or eat very little. If left to decide how much he eats, it will be less than ideal in the early days but increase gradually as he lets down his guard and becomes more relaxed while feeding.

I recommend that you use the night to boost baby's intake, but only enough to cover his basic needs in the short term. Too much at night can shift the balance from baby mostly eating in the day to mostly eating at night. While the volumes recommended below will be less than what baby needs on a daily basis, it's **only temporary** until he willingly starts to drink more while awake during the day.

Below 10 ounces (300 ml)

If your baby's milk intake during the day (six am to six pm or other 12-hour period) is below 10 ounces, which is possible on Days 1 to 3, offer him one or two feeds during the night in either an awake or sleepy state to ensure he reaches the 10-ounce minimum. **He can of course have more;** so don't stop the feed because he has reached 10 ounces. If he wakes later in the night and demands another feed, provide one.

If your baby rejects bottle-feeds while awake and asleep, offer milk from a syringe, medicine cup or sippy cup so that he reaches the 10-ounce minimum. Ensure baby is awake and in a fully upright position when providing milk by syringe or cup to prevent choking due to milk running to the back of his throat.

If your baby also breastfeeds, offer him at least two breastfeeds during the night. If he appears to be unsatisfied after breastfeeding then offer a bottle-feed in an awake or sleepy state.

Remember, you must not pressure him to feed while awake or asleep. Most parents find it's not difficult to ensure their baby receives the minimum of 10 ounces. If your baby gets **close** to 10 ounces of milk but has not quite made it, don't panic. You will probably find he does better on Day 2.

Note: 10 ounces is based on regular strength breast milk or formula – that is, 20 kcal per ounce or 67 kcal per 100 ml. If your baby is given high-energy feeds, milk intake could be a **little** lower so long as his total daily fluids are boosted to around 10 ounces with additional water.

If by chance your baby **completely rejects all feeds in the day** and he's way short of the 10-ounce minimum fluid intake by the end of the night, something I have not found occurs when a baby is healthy and able to feed, then return to your previous feeding methods, have baby checked by a doctor to make sure there's no underlying physical problem. Only attempt this process again if your healthcare professional thinks it's advisable and is available to help you monitor the situation.

Ten to 14 ounces (300–415 ml)

If your baby has taken 10–14 ounces of milk during the day, **offer** one night feed in an awake or sleepy state. Remember, 'offer' does not mean he must take it. **If he rejects** your offer, try again later in the night. If he rejects then, leave him to sleep. **If he accepts** a night feed, then provide a second feed only if he wakes to demand it. If he doesn't wake to demand a second night feed, leave him to sleep.

Fourteen+ ounces (415 ml+)

- **If baby is younger than six months,** offer one feed in the late evening (some time between nine pm and midnight) in an awake or sleepy state, and then allow him to wake and demand any additional night feeds. If he wakes and demands a second night feed, then provide one. Otherwise leave him sleeping.
- **If baby is over six months old,** he can be left to sleep through the night if he doesn't demand a night feed (after consuming more than 14 ounces in the day). If he wakes to demand one or more night feeds, provide these.
- **If baby is underweight,** offer one feed in the late evening either in an awake or sleepy state. If he rejects your offer of a night feed, don't worry. It means he will be all the more hungry the next day. If he wakes to demand one or more night feeds, provide these.

Please note: These figures apply to normal, physically well babies to cover basic needs of larger babies in the **short term**. This means smaller babies receive more in relation to body weight. These figures apply to regular-strength formula or breast milk.

If you have a **severely** underweight baby or special needs baby, please consult with his doctor regarding what would be an acceptable minimal daily intake on a short-term basis (a few days) and only attempt this behavioral approach to feeding management with his doctor's approval and supervision.

How to offer feeds

Demonstrate respect

Most babies who are averse to bottle-feeding have been repeatedly made to take the nipple into their mouth against their will. Imagine what it would feel like if someone tried to put food into your mouth without your permission. You would probably get annoyed or upset. What if they kept on doing it even after you told them to stop? You would undoubtedly become irate. This is because you can decide for yourself if you want food or not. So too can healthy babies. Once your baby is old enough to signal hunger and satisfaction, he can decide whether he will accept food when offered and how much he needs to eat. He will become angry or upset if you try to put the nipple into his mouth against his will.

To change your baby's negative feelings about feeding, this must stop. To regain his trust you need to demonstrate respect for his right to decide when and how much he will eat by 'asking' (though your actions) his permission to put the nipple into his mouth. I will explain.

How to seek permission

To give permission a baby needs to recognize the bottle. Whether a baby knows what a bottle is and connects it with satisfying his hunger depends on his memory and experiences bottle-feeding. Once he has made this connection he will indicate whether he wants the bottle or not by his behavior.

You 'ask' your baby's permission by showing him the bottle. Once he's in a feeding position, move the bottle into his line of sight, about six to eight inches (15–20 cm) in front of his face, and **pause** as you gauge his reaction. Some parents do this naturally, unaware that by checking baby's response they're asking baby's permission.

You can also ask him verbally if he wants the bottle as you pause. Doing so can be a good way to remind you that you need to gain his permission before putting the nipple into his mouth.

Of course your baby can't verbally give consent, but he can show you. Once he's seen the bottle he will give you permission to put the nipple into his mouth by indicating receptiveness, or deny permission by displaying signs of rejection. Signs that indicate receptiveness and rejection are described in Table 10.1.

Table 10.1: Receptiveness or rejection

Receptiveness	Rejection
<ul><li>looking at the bottle</li><li>getting excited by the sight of the bottle</li><li>opening his mouth to accept the bottle</li><li>grabbing the bottle to bring it to his mouth</li></ul>	<ul><li>clamping his mouth shut</li><li>turning head away or from side to side</li><li>pushing the bottle away or hitting the bottle</li><li>arching back</li></ul> **Note**: Baby could reject because he's not hungry or because he's averse to feeding. A baby who is averse to feeding will reject more intensely and may cry or scream at the sight of the bottle.

Under three months: Gauge response

A newborn baby could be crying due to hunger, see the bottle, but if he's not made the connection between the bottle and satisfying hunger, he's not going to indicate he wants it. Instead, he may continue to cry until the nipple is in his mouth.

I encourage you to still seek your newborn baby's permission because this will be a good habit to get into in preparation for the time when he will indicate if he wants it or not. However, if when you do this it appears like he doesn't recognize what the bottle means (a way to soothe his hunger), place the nipple into his mouth while he's crying and gauge his response. He will either start sucking, which means acceptance, or become upset, turn his head sharply to the side or arch back, in which case take this as a rejection.

If he shows signs of rejection, remove the bottle immediately. Be mindful that babies typically raise their tongue when crying. So take care to place the nipple over his tongue and not under.

If he's not crying when you offer him a feed and doesn't open his mouth upon seeing the bottle, try gently tapping or stroking his lips with the end of the nipple to see if this entices him to open his mouth. If he doesn't open his mouth to accept the bottle, he's not interested. Consider this as rejection. If he pulls away from the bottle in an upset manner, also take this as rejection.

Three+ months: Seek permission

If a bottle-fed baby is over three months old, and has had prior experience bottle-feeding, he can recognize a bottle and has learned to link this to feeding. Upon seeing the bottle he can decide if he wants it or not. From this age, you need to gain your baby's permission before placing the nipple into his mouth.

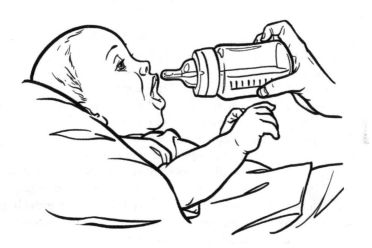

Baby is receptive

If he shows signs of receptiveness, he's giving permission; therefore, place the nipple into his mouth.

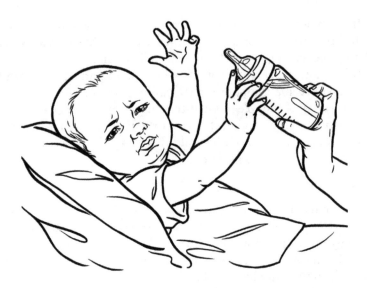

Baby rejects

If your baby displays signs of rejection, you don't have his permission; therefore, **don't** attempt to put the nipple into his mouth. Remove the bottle immediately, and say to him 'I can see you don't want to eat now. That's okay. You can eat later.' Or something along these lines.

Seeking your baby's permission, and accepting his rejection, may be quite different to what you have done in the past. You might have put the nipple into his mouth regardless of whether he indicated he wanted it or not. Saying the suggested words is more for you than your baby. Your actions will be enough for him. Saying these words reinforces into your subconscious that you're acknowledging that your baby doesn't want to eat right now, and that you're providing an appropriate response by removing the bottle. In time, responding in harmony with his cues will become automatic.

Expect rejections! Many babies who are averse to feeding will try to avoid feeding until ravenous. So just because your baby displays signs of hunger or because it's been many hours since he last fed, it doesn't mean he's going to accept your offer to feed him. He will, when he gets hungry enough. In the early days of resolving his aversion, he may need to get **really** hungry before he does.

Baby is distracted

If your baby is calm and not showing signs of receptiveness or rejection when presented with the bottle, he might be distracted. In this case, talk to him and gain his attention, or try gently tapping or stroking his lips with the end of the nipple. He will either open his mouth to accept the bottle or reject by pulling away. But don't do this if he has already shown signs of rejection.

How many times to offer at each feed

Your baby could reject your offer outright, perhaps quite forcefully in the early days, or he could take very little, stop sucking and suddenly become upset or distressed because he's anticipating being pressured. Or he could stop for other reasons, such as discomfort due to gastro-colic reflex (which triggers intestinal contractions causing baby to bear down like he wants to poop) or discomfort of intestinal contractions caused by the side effects of medications or because he wants to burp, or because he was distracted.

To reduce the risk that you might cut his feed short if he was to stop for a reason other than rejection, I recommend you offer twice at each feed, with a five-minute break between each offer. It doesn't need to be literally five minutes. It's just break to give him time to calm down. You can provide a longer break if you feel he's more receptive at the second offer as a result. However, I suggest the break be no longer than 20 minutes. An extensive break will at some point become the next feed. If he rejects or takes very little at the second offer, end the feed.

You're going to feel tempted to offer repeatedly. Please don't. He might take it due to coercion or pressure, which could reinforce his aversion. Or it might anger him to be repeatedly offered the bottle when he's already rejected twice. So I encourage you to end the feed after the second offer. He will be offered food again soon enough.

Around five percent of babies become irritated as a result of being offered again (a second time) after they reject the feed. So if you find your baby accepts the first offer but repeatedly gets upset and rejects the second, then offer only once.

How to respond to baby's cues

For a baby to want to eat and continue eating for long enough to reach the point of feeling full, he needs to associate feeding with something that is pleasing and satisfying. The most effective way to help your baby feel this way is to respond according to his feeding cues. Table 10.2 lists signs that indicate baby wants to continue or stop feeding.

Table 10.2: Baby wants to continue or stop

Baby wants to continue	Baby wants to stop
• continues to suck • holds bottle in his mouth while he pauses	• stops sucking • rolls his tongue around the nipple without sucking • pushes the nipple out of his mouth with his tongue • pushes the bottle away with his hands or hits the bottle • turns his head sharply to the side in a tense manner • arches back **Note:** Baby could stop in a passive way when hunger is satisfied or in an upset, tense manner due to being averse to feeding

... while baby feeds

Observe your baby's feeding behavior and follow his lead. While he's happy to suck, let him. Don't break the feed to burp, change his position or mop up a dribble of milk. He will let you know if something is bothering him. Don't rock or bounce him while he's feeding. This might cause him to lose suction and frustrate him.

Engage in eye contact with him while feeding, if he will let you. Talk to him or sing to him as he feeds. It doesn't need to be incessant talking or signing. Observe his reaction to your gaze and voice. If this soothes him and allows him to remain focused on feeding, continue. But if it distracts or upsets him, ease off.

... whether he wants lots or a little

Remember your baby gets to decide how much he will drink. Anything he drinks must be on his terms, not yours. Suppress the urge you may be feeling to control his feeds and don't try to make him drink if he doesn't want to.

Watch for signs that indicate that he wants to stop, and respond accordingly by removing the bottle. If he tries to push the nipple out of his mouth with his tongue or hands, turns his head sharply to the side or arches back to break away from the bottle, let him. Don't try to make him keep the nipple in his mouth and don't try to prevent him from breaking away by following him with the bottle. Allow him to turn away. (**Note:** This is different to a relaxed baby turning his head to look around while continuing to suck, which is not rejection. In this case you can follow him with the bottle.)

If he stops feeding and becomes tense or upset at that point, take a five-minute break and reoffer. If he rejects or indicates he wants to stop at the second offer, end the feed.

Babies who are averse to feeding usually only willingly drink small amounts before rejecting. So don't expect your baby to eat until satisfaction in the early days. Avoid tactics to 'encourage' him to drink more because you know he's not eaten enough and your anxiety levels are high. Such tactics typically involve gentle forms of pressure.

... pauses, burps or distractions

A baby can and will display behavior while feeding that might disrupt the feed without rejecting the feed.

- **If he wants to pause,** let him. Allow him to set the pace. Don't jiggle or twist the bottle to try to make him start again. When a baby is pausing he's relaxed, not tense and upset.
- **If he stops to burp,** this is not a rejection. Burp him and reoffer the bottle, but seek his permission before putting the nipple back into his mouth.
- **If he gets distracted by something,** this is not a rejection. Gain his attention and reoffer.
- **If he accidently knocks** the nipple out of his mouth, this is not a rejection. Reoffer.

... if in doubt

At times you'll be unsure whether your baby is rejecting or not. This is probably because he's unsure too. He's expecting to be pressured to feed and it's not happening. So he's confused. He remembers being pressured, so he's on edge. Is it going to happen? Is it safe to feed? He sucks tentatively, but he's half expecting to be hassled so he stops feeding and wants to get away before that happens, therefore he's sending mixed signals. He will give clearer signals once he's learned to trust he's not going to be pressured.

In the meantime, if you're in doubt about what his behavior means, then go for a break or end the feed. Better to stop too soon than risk causing him to feel pressured. If he actually did want the bottle at the time, but you removed it, it won't take him long to figure out that he needs to take it when it's offered without messing about. He's not going to starve during the short break he may need to wait before being offered another feed.

You may be surprised by how quickly baby learns. Lucas, aged four-and-a-half months, was sending mixed messages and so his mother would remove the bottle and go for a break or end the feed. Within a day, he started to grasp the bottle. It was his way of saying, 'Don't take it away, I am not done yet.' It still took many days for him to enjoy eating, but at least his mom could now read his clearer signals. Not all babies will grasp the bottle. So don't expect your baby to do this.

You probably have questions about different scenarios at this point. I encourage you to keep reading. In the next chapter you will find answers to frequently asked questions about feeding.

Feeding FAQs

> I plan to follow your feeding recommendations
> but I am afraid I will do something wrong that
> will stop Imogen from getting over her aversion.
> – Bridget

Bridget – like most parents – had many questions about how she might handle different scenarios. Babies react differently to my feeding recommendations depending on the habits they have already established. I'll describe the main reactions here – like not showing hunger, screaming, and falling asleep – and how I recommend you to respond. I'll also look at other scenarios, like when baby wants to hold the bottle or when she doesn't want to be held to feed, or wants movement.

What if baby doesn't show hunger?

When I advise parents to wait until their baby shows signs of hunger before offering a feed, some say they don't know what this looks like. They claim they have never seen their baby display hunger before. They express concerns that unlike other babies, their baby might not feel hunger.

In many cases I suspect that baby has not ever felt hunger due to parents' diligence in feeding her at preset times and making sure she ate a prescribed amount. But a healthy baby might not give clear signals of hunger for other reasons:

- Some babies have such easy-going temperaments they signal hunger in a very subdued way and don't complain if feeds are delayed.
- A baby with feeding aversion will try to avoid feeding and therefore may not show typical cues of hunger.
- Appetite can be suppressed when a baby is **severely** underweight.

Once parents stop trying to make their baby feed against her will, most babies will start to display behavioral cues that indicate hunger within a day or two.

While your baby is getting over her feeding aversion, if she **doesn't show signs of hunger** offer her a feed around three hours after her previous feed. Offer a feed sooner if she shows signs of hunger sooner. But let her go longer if she's napping at three hours. Don't wake her to feed her during the day.

Once she's over her aversion and willingly taking good volumes of milk, then allow her to demand feeds rather than offer at three hours. You may find she is content to go longer than three hours without eating once her milk intake increases.

What if baby rejected or took little, when do I offer again?

The recommendations described in Chapter 10 using a cue- and time-based approach apply regardless of how much your baby takes or whether she takes anything at all.

What if baby looks like she wants it again after rejecting?

Conflicted feeding behavior – where baby takes a few sips, pulls away, wants it again, takes a few sip, pulls away etc and appears like she's wavering between wanting to eat and not wanting to eat – is common in the case of an unresolved feeding aversion. Following my advice to respond to baby's cues it would make sense to keep giving it to her while she wants it, right? After all, there's no pressure involved. Well, there are exceptions to each rule (except the 'no-pressure' rule) and this is one of them.

Based on my experience, I have found that if the parent returns the bottle time and time again, this tends to reinforce baby's conflicted feeding behavior. So weeks down the track baby is still feeding in this tense, disjointed fashion, and her total daily milk volume – though better than before – is not as high as it could be. It's as if her feeding aversion is only partially resolved.

If your baby displays conflicted feeding behavior, I recommend you remove the bottle when she breaks away, turns her head or arches back **in a tense upset manner,** indicating rejection. Then go for a break before offering a second time or end the feed if this occurs at the second offer. This might sound like punishment for rejection. But its purpose is to avoid accidently reinforcing conflicted feeding behavior. By removing the bottle you're clearly demonstrating to your baby that you're not going to pressure her to eat.

If the bottle is not there when she returns, she will quickly learn to **not** break away when hungry. You might be surprised at how quickly she figures out that she had better eat when a bottle is offered or remain hungry for a little longer (which might be five minutes until the second offer, or one hour or less until the next feed if she's showing signs of hunger at that time). As a result, the volume of milk she takes each feed will start to increase within one or two feeds, and continue to increase over many days (with ups and downs).

While it might feel like you're starving your baby by removing the bottle when she's willing to reattach, you're ultimately encouraging greater enjoyment in feeding over the long term. She's not going to starve as a result of waiting a while to be offered again.

What if baby screams *before* seeing the bottle?

Some babies who have become averse to feeding will start screaming as soon as they are laid in a feeding position or when a bib is placed around their neck because they know this signals they're about to be fed.

Show your baby the bottle, determine whether she shows signs of receptiveness or rejection and follow the recommendations on how to offer a feed in Chapter 10.

If you suspect her screaming is mostly because she recognizes she's about to be fed, try feeding her in a different place to where you would usually feed her. Or a different feeding position, one that she doesn't normally associate with feeding, for example while facing out. As she demonstrates that she is more relaxed (which will occur while getting over her aversion) then decide if you would like her to return her to a normal feeding position.

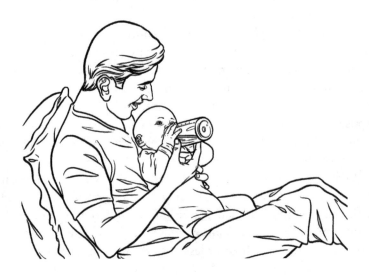

What if baby gets drowsy or falls asleep while feeding?

Some babies who are averse to feeding feed better when drowsy or asleep compared to when awake because they're not as aware of what's happening. Or they may have learned to rely on feeding as a way to fall asleep. Whatever the reason, sleep-feeding can delay or prevent your baby from learning to enjoy feeding while awake.

I recommend you avoid feeding her in a drowsy state or while she's sleeping during the day. And ultimately at night also. However, avoiding feeding in a drowsy or sleepy state at night may need to be achieved in a progressive way. There are exceptions to the 'no sleep-feeding' rule at night. (See Chapter 10 for details.)

... during the day

If your baby becomes drowsy while feeding, prompt her to remain awake. Talk to her, stroke her, give her a break to burp her, or change her diaper as a way to awaken her, and offer again. (You can offer straight away as she did not reject the feed.) If you can't keep her awake, end the feed, even if she seems willing to keep sucking while drowsy. The more she drinks in a sleepy state the longer she will be able to hold out before accepting a feed while awake. Feeding her in a sleepy state could mean she holds out until next naptime and then once again falls asleep while feeding. She might get by feeding at each nap, but it won't solve her aversion or encourage her to feed while awake.

... during the night

The more milk your baby drinks at night the less she needs to drink during the day. Feeding a sleeping baby can encourage night feeds that a baby might not need. And by doing so shift the balance from mostly feeding in the day to mostly feeding at night.

There are three exceptions to the 'no sleep-feed' rule at night. Sleep feeds might be provided in the following instances:

1. To ensure a baby reaches the minimum of 10 ounces (300 ml) in a 24-hour period.

2. If an underweight baby does not wake to demand night feeds.

3. If your baby is younger than six months of age, you might prefer to give **one** sleep-feed (also called dream feed) in the late evening.

Apart from these few exceptions, as a **general** guide, aim for your baby to wake and demand night feeds and for her to start any feeds at night while she's awake. If she becomes drowsy while feeding during the night allow her to continue sucking until she stops. This also involves a compromise from the 'no sleep-feed' rule. The reason is because she needs milk in her belly in order to sleep. If she's not sleeping, you're not sleeping, and neither of you will cope well the following day. But reserve this for night feeds only.

These compromises relate to the **adjustment phase** (the time it takes to resolve her feeding aversion). **Once your baby is no longer averse to feeding,** you may need to avoid sleep-feeding at night to improve the quality or her sleep (explained in Chapter 12) and to encourage a normal day-night feeding pattern which means baby mostly eats during the day.

Should I give baby water?

It's okay to offer baby water. However, not from a bottle, not directly before a bottle-feed, and not too much.

Let her learn that the bottle contains milk that satisfies her hunger. Offer water from a spoon, syringe, medicine cup or sippy cup rather than a bottle. When you offer your baby water, have her in a fully upright position so water doesn't fall to the back of her throat and trigger her gag reflex or cause choking. When providing water your job is to offer, not to make your baby drink. It's up to her whether she wants to drink water or not.

Avoid offering water directly before bottle-feeds. If your baby's tummy contains water, she may be less inclined to accept milk or drink less than she would have otherwise.

Your baby will possibly reject offers of water or drink only small amounts. If by chance she does want to drink large amounts, eg 4 ounces (120 ml) or more **over the course of the day**, check with your healthcare professional that she's not drinking too much water.

Should I provide encouragement?

No doubt you will be celebrating on the inside when you see your baby willingly feeding after enduring weeks or months of stress as a result of her feeding aversion. And you will want to encourage this. However, positive reinforcement such as clapping, cheering, telling baby she's a good girl or that she's doing a great job because she's sucking, is not necessary. Feeding and eating are normal daily activities that your baby will do every day for the rest of her life. Her willingness to feed is **not** exceptional – even though it might feel that way – and therefore not something that requires celebration.

Your baby doesn't require celebration to motivate her to feed. Having her hunger satisfied, enjoyment in the taste and experiences associated with feeding and eating in a social environment with her mom, dad or other caregiver engaging with her and responding appropriately to her cues is encouragement enough.

What if baby wants movement while feeding?

Feeding your baby while you stand and rock, bounce on a yoga ball or walk around with her in your arms is not practical over the long term. At some point she'll get too big and heavy for you to comfortably hold while feeding her. Plus it may be difficult to feed her in this way in public and so it could limit your family's freedom to enjoy outings.

Start this process by feeding her in the way you wish her to feed over the long-term. She might complain and resist feeding a little longer at the start because you're not standing, rocking or bouncing her as she has learned to expect, but she will come around. You just have to be consistent in offering her feeds while you are seated and stationary.

What if baby doesn't want to be held while feeding?

Not wanting to be held in a feeding position in the parent's arms is common when baby is averse to feeding.

As a baby's memory develops she learns to link a sequence of events. When she's held in a feeding position, she thinks she's about to be fed. If past feeding experiences have been stressful, she might start to fuss or cry, even when there's no bottle in sight, simply because she's anticipating being pressured to feed. My recommendation varies depending on baby's age.

Younger than eight months

If your baby is younger than eight months, I recommend you persist offering her feeds while she's in your arms despite her resistance. She will come around to accepting a feed while in your arms when she gets hungry enough. She will probably be tense and cautious for many days, expecting you to pressure her as you've done in the past, but provided you respond to her cues without any pressure she will gradually relax and ultimately enjoy feeding while in your arms.

Learning to enjoy feeding time in your arms will make it easier for you to feed her outside your home, as opposed to her only wanting to feed in a specific place.

If you choose to feed her elsewhere, say in a rocker, baby buggy or stroller, baby seat or propped on cushions, she might accept the bottle sooner, but she may then continue to reject feeding in your arms over the long term. But the choice is yours! Your baby can get over her bottle-feeding aversion while feeding in or out of your arms. Most parents having suffered long-term stress associated with an infant feeding aversion are happy that their baby willingly feeds and don't mind if she feeds elsewhere.

Eight+ months

If your baby is older than eight months, attempt to feed her in your arms to show her you will respond to her cues, but if she gets upset, allow her to feed elsewhere, if this is what she prefers. Babies begin to exert their independence while feeding around eight months of age. Even babies without a feeding aversion sometimes prefer to feed independently.

Consistency is key!

Whatever decision you make about your baby's feeding position, be consistent. Choose what you feel will work best and stick with it. Trying too many positions during the adjustment phase could cause her greater frustration than sticking to the one. That doesn't mean you can't ever deviate from this position, but consistency minimizes needless frustration while resolving her aversion.

What if baby wants to hold the bottle?

If baby wants to hold the bottle, let her. Most babies, even those without a feeding aversion, want to hold their own bottles from around eight months or sooner. Babies who have been pressured to feed in the past may be more willing to feed if they're allowed to control the bottle.

If your baby indicates she wants to hold the bottle but doesn't yet have the coordination required, consider purchasing handles that attach to the bottle to help her.

What if baby pulls the bottle in and out of her mouth?

If baby pulls the bottle in and out of her mouth, let her. She's testing her newfound ability to control the feed. She's possibly never experienced the freedom to do this before and she's fascinated by this new development. The novelty will wear off in a few days and she will stop.

What if baby starts playing with the bottle and not feeding?

If baby starts playing with the bottle, let her – within reason. Give her two or three minutes to see if she's just being cautious before starting to feed. However, if she's not feeding after a couple of minutes, she's obviously not hungry enough to want to feed. In this case, end the feed and try again later.

Playing with the bottle without feeding is not a habit you want to encourage. She could be playing with so many other far more interesting things.

Getting enough sleep is essential to baby's success when it comes to getting over a feeding aversion. Next I will explain how to support your baby's sleep during this process.

12
Support baby's sleep

> I have to feed Liam while he's sleeping now because it's the only way I can get him to drink enough. Sometimes he wakes up and won't eat and then won't go back to sleep. Then I have a grouchy, tired and hungry baby to cope with. I know he's not getting enough sleep, but my priority has been getting him to feed. I really need to fix his feeding issues so we can all have a normal life. – Lara

I agree with Lara; resolving Liam's feeding issues is more important than fixing any sleeping problem he might have. However, a tired baby may not eat well. If Liam is not getting enough sleep this could make it more difficult to resolve his feeding aversion.

Based on my experience, nine out of 10 babies who are averse to feeding also have a sleeping problem that causes sleep deprivation to varying degrees. It's typically assumed that baby is not sleeping well because of hunger. While this can be a reason, often other causes are involved. I will describe these in this chapter.

It's usually not practical to resolve a baby's sleeping problem until he's over his feeding aversion. However, there may be steps you can take in the short-term to minimize sleep deprivation, and the negative impact it may have on your baby's feeding. Once he's eating well, you may find his sleep improves, or discover that you need to turn your attention towards resolving his sleeping issues.

Why is sleep important?

We all know that if a baby doesn't feed well, he's not going to sleep well. But the reverse applies equally. When a baby is not getting enough sleep his frustration tolerance will be low or non-existent. He could reject your offer to feed, fuss throughout the feed, or fall asleep while feeding. Therefore, supporting your baby to get the amount of sleep he needs could have a positive influence on his acceptance of feeds and milk intake.

How much sleep do babies need?

During the time it takes to resolve your baby's feeding aversion your task is to minimize his sleep debt. Sleep debt is the difference between the amount of sleep he needs and the amount he gets. Knowing how much sleep is average for a baby of his age may help you estimate how much sleep he needs.

Table 12.1: Average number of hours sleep for age

Age	Average total sleep time (hours)	Average night sleep (hours)	Average day sleep (hours)
1 week	16½	8½	8
1 month	15½	8¾	6¾
3 months	15	10	5
6 months	14¼	11	3¼
9 months	14	11¼	2¾
12 months	13¾	11¾	2

Some babies need more or less sleep than average, so please use the table above as a rough estimation. If your baby is content, it doesn't matter how much sleep he's getting. But if he's often cranky and also **not** getting close to average sleep for his age, then lack of sleep could be contributing to his bad mood, as it does for us all. The next step is to identify the reason or reasons he may be missing sleep.

Why baby might lack sleep

A baby could be lacking sleep for many different reasons. In cases where babies are troubled by a feeding aversion the top reasons include:

1. hunger

2. dependence on negative sleep associations

3. tiredness cues are overlooked or mistaken as hunger, boredom or pain

4. disrupted sleep due to sleep-feeding

5. developmental changes

6. physical or medical problems.

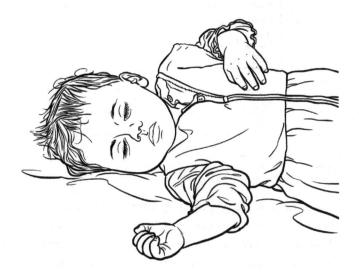

For some babies, lack of sleep can be due to a combination of two or three of these reasons. I will explain how these problems could adversely affect your baby's sleep while resolving his feeding aversion, and what to do to minimize his sleep debt.

Note: The order of these sleep deficit causes is different for babies who are **not** averse to feeding.

Hunger complications

To resolve your baby's feeding aversion, it's vital that you allow him to decide when he will eat and how much he's willing to take. During the early stages of the adjustment phase, a time when he's going to still have negative feelings about feeding, his milk intake will be low. At times he'll be upset due to hunger. And yet, despite feeling the discomfort of hunger he might not be willing to eat. And when he does, he probably won't eat enough to feel content. So this means the likelihood of sleep disturbance due to hunger will be high.

Ensuring your baby has sufficient sleep is going to be tricky in the first three to five days. As best you try, it's simply not going to be possible to support him to get the perfect amount of sleep. At times his feelings of hunger and tiredness will collide. When this happens, tiredness tends to dominate. As a result, he's less likely to eat, and he may find it difficult to fall asleep and stay asleep due to hunger. Naps will likely be short.

As your baby learns to trust that he's no longer going to be pressured to eat, his milk intake will slowly increase, and provided there's no underlying sleep problem – which there could be – it will become easier to get him to fall asleep and his naps will extend. In the meantime, all you can do is manage the sleep situation as best you can while following my feeding recommendations, and try to remain patient until the situation improves.

If he has an underlying sleeping problem, this is likely to be due to learned dependence on negative sleep associations. In this case, his sleeping won't necessarily improve as his milk intake increases.

Dependence on negative sleep associations

Sleep associations are the conditions, props or activities a baby learns to rely on as a way to fall sleep. Babies typically learn to rely on one or more of the following sleep associations:

- Physical contact with a parent or caregiver; eg, cuddles in a parent's arms, laying on a parent's chest or next to a parent while bed sharing, or carried in a sling.
- Feeding to sleep (breast or bottle).
- Being patted, stroked, jiggled or bounced.
- Rocked in a baby rocker, bouncer, swing, hammock or stroller.
- Movement while driven in a car.
- Swaddled or dressed in a baby sleep sack.
- Music, radio, white noise, womb-like sounds, or shushing.
- Sucking on a pacifier.
- Clutching a security blanket or soft toy.

Sleep associations can be divided into two categories; positive and negative.

Positive versus negative sleep associations

Positive sleep associations are present as baby first falls asleep and **remain present** throughout baby's entire sleep. For example, falling asleep while in his bed (bassinette or crib), swaddling or infant sleep sack, thumb and finger sucking (baby's not your's) and security objects like a lovey.

Negative sleep associations are present at the time baby falls asleep but **are absent or change** in some way after baby has fallen asleep. This can include anything you do to actively assist your baby to fall asleep if you remove your help once he's asleep. It also includes props or sleep aids such as a pacifier, swing, musical mobile or others that fall out or switch off after baby has fallen asleep.

How sleep associations affect sleep

Sleep associations have a profound effect on a baby's ability to sleep. The presence or absence of a baby's sleep associations can influence how easily he falls asleep and whether he remains asleep long enough to have his sleep needs met or wakes too soon.

Falling asleep

Unlike you, your baby cannot take himself off to bed and set up his environment and sleep associations when he's ready to sleep. He relies on you or another caregiver to do this for him. Once he has learned to associate certain conditions with sleeping, when tired he will fuss and cry for his sleep associations to be provided. If they are made available to him, he will drop off to sleep relatively quickly (provided he's not hungry).

However, if his sleep associations are withheld, perhaps because you overlooked his signs of tiredness or misinterpreted his tired signs as hunger, boredom or pain, or because you were unaware that he has learned to rely on certain sleep associations to fall asleep, he may remain awake despite his readiness to sleep. The longer he's denied his sleep associations, the more tired he becomes, the more he fusses, and the greater the risk he will reach the point of distress due to overtiredness.

Remaining asleep

The presence of a baby's familiar sleep associations don't just help him to fall asleep, they also support him to remain asleep for as long as he needs to wake refreshed. He might wake sooner if a physical need – like hunger – requires attention, but the risk of him waking too soon is significantly reduced if his sleep associations remain consistent throughout his entire sleep.

If your baby's sleep associations are absent or change in some way after he falls asleep, he's at increased risk of waking prematurely from his sleep. But only if he notices the change. He's probably not going to notice the loss of his sleep associations while he's in a deep sleep stage of a sleep cycle, but when he next enters into light sleep he might. He's likely to wake if he senses a change to his sleep associations. If he has not had enough sleep, he will either wake cranky or quickly become that way owing to tiredness.

How this changes according to level of fatigue

Once a baby has learned to rely on particular sleep associations, he may resist falling asleep and wake too soon without them. When sleep is delayed or broken owing to the absence of his sleep associations, this can cause a sleep debt. If this occurs a number of times throughout the day, his sleep debt will accumulate. By the evening he could reach the point of overtiredness. Once overtired, his little body will start to release stress hormones that make it difficult for him to fall asleep, even if his sleep associations are present at that time.

After what could be many hours of fussing and crying due to the stress associated with overtiredness, eventually he falls asleep as physical exhaustion overpowers him. Once asleep, a newborn baby might remain asleep for an extended time, too exhausted to notice or care if his sleep associations are present or not, and in some cases too exhausted to wake to demand night feeds. Whereas a baby over the age of four months might wake multiple times during the night if his sleep associations are missing.

Feeding-sleep association

Definition

Feeding-sleep association means baby has learned to depend on feeding as a way to fall sleep. He then wants to feed when he's tired. But he won't necessarily be hungry at the time.

Sleep-feeding is when a baby feeds while drowsy or during sleep. Baby might become tired while feeding and doze off or the parent might choose to feed their baby after he has fallen asleep because he resists less. Baby is not necessarily dependent on feeding as a way to fall asleep. If he is, he also has a feeding-sleep association.

Of the many sleep associations a baby could learn to rely on, I single out feeding to sleep. The combination of **feeding aversion and feeding-sleep association** is one of the most challenging to turn around.

Many babies who have a feeding aversion also have a sleeping problem. Both have the potential to **indirectly** affect each other; however, in most cases these are separate problems. In these cases, I encourage parents to tackle each problem separately – feeding aversion first, sleeping problem second. However, in the case of a feeding aversion where baby also has feeding-sleep association, the two problems are **directly linked**. Feeding a baby during sleep reinforces his sleeping problem and also removes motivation for him to want to eat while awake.

Following my 'no sleep-feeding' rule means parents may need to make changes to the way their baby is settled to sleep **at the same time** as they resolve his feeding aversion. This can be achieved, but it's going to mean extra crankiness on baby's part and extra stress for parents in the early days as baby learns to fall asleep in a new way at a time that his milk intake is likely to be low.

Solutions to sleep association problems

To resolve a sleeping problem related to dependence on negative sleep associations means changing a baby's sleep associations from those that require others' help or unreliable props (negative sleep associations) to those that support independent settling (positive sleep associations). This can be achieved through sleep training.

However, I **don't** recommend you attempt sleep training while helping your baby get over his feeding aversion. Resolving his feeding aversion is going to be unsettling for him and you in the short term due to hunger complications. Trying to deal with both problems at the same time would needlessly cause more stress for all involved, and may result in failure on both fronts. Focus on what's most important, and that is his feeding aversion. In the interim, you can support his sleep in a number of ways.

How to support baby's sleep

My recommendations on how to support your baby's sleep differ depending on whether he's in the process of having his feeding aversion resolved or whether he's no longer averse to feeding.

While resolving baby's aversion

If you're still resolving baby's feeding aversion you might help baby gain more sleep in a few ways. First identify your baby's current sleep associations and provide these when you observe his tiredness cues. This will help him to fall asleep.

If he often wakes after napping only briefly, decide if you can encourage more sleep by **returning** his sleep associations. Or consider whether it may be more effective to **maintain** his sleep associations throughout his entire sleep.

Returning baby's sleep associations usually works at night but might not get him back to sleep if his naps are cut short and he wakes crying. By then he could be too upset owing to the loss of his sleep associations to return to sleep.

If you were to return his sleep associations **as he arouses** between sleep cycles and before he wakes fully, there's a better chance of getting him to return to sleep. For example, if he's accustomed to being rocked to sleep in his crib while sucking a pacifier, you may need to observe him closely as he naps. When you see him begin to stir between sleep cycles make sure he has his pacifier and rock him back into deep sleep. Of course this won't work if he's already had enough sleep.

Maintaining his sleep associations. If he continues to be troubled by short naps, you may need to maintain his sleep associations throughout his entire sleep ... if possible. For example, if he's reliant on being cuddled to sleep in your arms, you may need to continue to cuddle him until he wakes.

An exception to continuing to provide your baby's current sleep association is if he is reliant on feeding as a way to fall asleep. **In the case of a feeding-sleep association,** I recommend you not only avoid feeding your baby in a drowsy state (during the day but not necessarily at night) but that you also prevent him from falling asleep while sucking on a bottle, day and night. Remember: if during daytime feeds he becomes drowsy while feeding, talk to him, stroke him, break the feed, sit him up, wake him up and offer again. If you can't keep him awake, remove the bottle and end the feed. At night continue to feed him while drowsy but aim to prevent him from falling asleep while feeding. Change his diaper after the feed as a way to arouse him. Then settle him to sleep in a different way.

The aim is to simply avoid feeding him to sleep, not sleep train. If he likes to suck on a pacifier, you might give him this and cuddle him to sleep instead. There will be some resistance on his part for a few days owing to the change. But if you're consistent in not letting him fall asleep while feeding and instead settle him in the new way, it should get easier after around three days and nights.

After resolving baby's aversion

Once your baby's feeding issues are resolved, decide whether you wish to continue to support his sleep by providing his current sleep associations. If doing so 24/7 is not sustainable over the long-term, I recommend you consider sleep training. You will find various ways to manage or resolve sleep association problems in my infant sleep book – *Your Sleepless Baby* – available through my two websites **www.babycareadvice.com** and **www.yourbabyseries.com** as well as popular online book distributors.

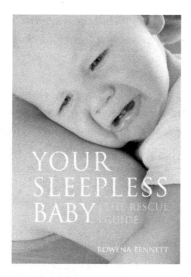

Overlooking baby's tired signs

Your baby can't tell you when he's ready to sleep but he will display signs that he is becoming agitated when tired. As his caregiver, it's up to you to recognize when he's tired and provide him with an opportunity to sleep.

Birth to three months

Young babies **rarely** display the typical signs of tiredness of children and adults. This is because of their body movements are primarily controlled by reflexes (a reflex is an automatic, involuntary response). Behavior commonly displayed by babies younger than three months of age that indicate tiredness, starting from early, subtle behavior to not-so subtle behavior, include:

- whining → crying → screaming
- glazed stare → looking away → turning head away (babies cannot turn their head away until about two months) → back arching (usually not until around three months)
- frowning → facial grimacing (a pained looking expression which involves tightly shut eyes and an open mouth)
- tightly clenched fists
- pulling up knees
- waving arms and legs → jerking, quick arm and leg movements
- seeking comfort by sucking or feeding.

If baby regularly falls asleep while bottle-feeding, it may mean he's developed a feeding-sleep association. In this case, he might appear as if he's hungry when he's tired.

Over three months

By three months of age many of baby's infant reflexes have disappeared and he has gained greater voluntary control over his arm and leg movements. So now he no longer frantically flails his arms and legs when you lay him down. Behavioral cues that indicate tiredness are easier to recognize in this age group compared to newborns. These include:

- whining → crying → screaming
- loss of interest in toys or playing
- turning head away → back arching
- sucking on fingers or hands
- pulling ears or hair
- rubbing nose or eyes
- yawning
- clinginess
- temper outbursts.

Just like adults, most babies do not yawn when they're tired. So if you're waiting to observe a yawn before settling baby to sleep, you could be leaving it too late.

Not all babies display the same signs or to the same intensity. Depending on their temperament (inborn personality traits), some babies may only display subtle signs of tiredness, whereas others may appear to go from content to distraught in a flash. But in reality most will display the subtle early signs of tiredness.

When to expect tiredness cues

In addition to learning what behavioral cues to watch for, you may find it helpful to know when to anticipate your baby is likely to become tired. Next you'll find the average daytime periods spent awake before needing a nap. During the night you don't want to encourage any time awake, other than that required for feeding.

Table 12.2: Average awake time for age

Age	Estimated awake during day (including feed)
2–6 weeks	1–1¼ hours
6 weeks–3 months	1–2 hours
3–6 months	2.0–2.5 hours
6–9 months	2.5–3 hours
9–12 months	3–4 hours

Consider the timeframe relevant for baby's age but watch for early signs of tiredness before trying to settle him off to sleep. If the timing is right and you notice signs that baby is becoming unsettled, you can feel fairly confident that tiredness is the reason, or at least partly responsible for his behavior.

When a baby is averse to feeding, and therefore not drinking as much as he needs, or if he has a sleep-association problem, sleep may be broken and so he may show signs of tiredness before the suggested time.

When he displays tiredness cues, check that his physical needs are met, take him into a quiet environment and settle him to sleep. He will settle quicker if you provide his familiar sleep associations at this time.

Disrupted sleep due to sleep-feeding

Parents sometimes find they accidentally wake their baby by their attempts to feed baby during sleep. If you follow my 'no sleep-feeding' rule this will no longer be a reason for your baby to lack sleep.

Developmental changes

As your baby matures and develops physically, emotionally and intellectually, he will undergo developmental changes that can affect his sleep. For example:

Brain development: Your baby will become increasingly more aware of his surroundings with age. As his memory develops, he will learn to expect a certain response from you and anticipate a sequence of events based on the care you have provided in the past. He will be able to recognize consistencies and inconsistencies in the care he receives. This includes the way he is settled to sleep.

Four months is a common age for babies' sleep to deteriorate. (This is often referred to as 'four month sleep regression'.) The most frequent cause is because of a baby's increased awareness of the absence of familiar sleep associations during light sleep. If he notices his sleep associations are missing, he's likely to wake still tired after one sleep cycle, and wake frequently during the night and cry out for his sleep associations to be returned. (A sleep cycle during the day can range from 20 to 45 minutes depending on age. The younger the baby, the shorter the sleep cycle.)

Emotional development means he will experience separation anxiety starting around seven months and peaking around nine to 10 months. He may start to wake and cry in the night to be reassured by your presence.

Physical development, such as rolling, sitting and standing, means your baby might practice these skills during what would normally be brief arousals between sleep cycles. He may then find himself stuck in a position he's unable to get out of without help. Upset by his predicament, he cries for help, and so a brief arousal becomes a full awakening that requires greater effort to return to sleep.

Provided there are no behavioral reasons for sleep disturbance, such as dependence on negative sleep associations, wakefulness due to developmental reasons is usually only temporary. Your baby will outgrow it.

Physical and medical conditions

Just like feeding issues, physical problems are last on the list when it comes to sleep problems affecting **physically well** babies. Of course, if a baby is ill or has an **untreated** condition that causes discomfort, the risk of a medical problem causing broken sleep shoots to the top of the list of possibilities.

Minor physical problems might include teething or constipation. More serious problems include illness, untreated digestive disorder, chronic conditions, and neurological impairment. Not only can these problems affect sleep, they could also negatively affect a baby's appetite and his desire or ability to eat.

If your baby has a physical problem, then ensure this is treated **before** starting my feeding recommendations. However, unrelated physical problems have the potential to occur **after** starting. If your baby experiences a physical problem while you're helping him get over his aversion to bottle-feeding, you need to weigh up how serious the problem is, whether it can it be quickly treated, and how close he is to being over his aversion.

Stopping the process before baby's aversion is resolved means he won't be willingly consuming sufficient amounts of milk. This might cause you to feel inclined to once again pressure him to eat or return to feeding him during sleep. In doing so, any progress already achieved may be lost. On the other hand, there is a point where it could be unreasonable to continue if he's ill.

If it's a case of teething or constipation, this can usually be managed or corrected quickly and you may find he's fine to continue. Note: My feeding recommendations don't usually cause a baby to become constipated. However, if a baby is prone to constipation he could become so during this process.

The following signs could indicate illness or a physical problem:

- fever
- vomiting
- diarrhea
- coughing, rattly chest, nasal discharge
- rashes
- persistent, inconsolable screaming unrelated to feeding times
- lethargy.

If your baby displays any of these signs, have him examined by a doctor. Check with his doctor whether it's advisable to continue with the feeding plan or return to previous feeding practices until he's well, at which time consider trying again to resolve his feeding aversion.

In the next chapter I will explain how to monitor your baby's progress throughout the process of resolving his aversion.

13
Monitor baby's progress

> It's Day 3 and Molly seems to be improving. She
> now takes the bottle when I offer but she's not
> drinking much. I'm worried she won't start taking
> more. When can I expect her to drink more? How
> will I know when she's over her feeding aversion?
> – Andrea

Andrea's feeling nervous, and for good reason; an infant feeding
aversion is one of the most stressful situations a parent can face. By
following my feeding recommendations Andrea will be taking a leap
of faith. She's now allowing Molly to decide the amount of milk she
will take. But this is new to Andrea, and is undoubtedly a daunting
prospect. If Andrea is not aware of what to expect, there's a high risk
that anxiety related to Molly's milk intake could cause her to give up
too soon, and revert back to her previous practice of pressuring Molly
to eat.

In this chapter I describe how babies typically behave in response
to my feeding recommendations. Knowing what to expect might lessen
your anxiety and help you feel more confident that things are on track.
That way, you can continue for long enough to achieve the ultimate
goal of your baby enjoying eating.

How long will this take?

I would love to provide desperate parents with an immediate remedy to their baby's feeding aversion without unsettling baby or parents in the short term, but no such solution exists. Patterns of behavior take time to establish, and they also take time to change.

A baby doesn't go from fearing to embracing feeding overnight. Even after parents cease all forms of pressure and respond in harmony with baby's cues, it can take weeks before she gets over a feeding aversion.

While the average time to resolve a feeding aversion using my **Five Steps to Success** is two weeks, it can vary depending on a baby's age, temperament, sensitivity to pressure, how often and for how long baby has been pressured to feed, and the level of pressure applied (eg, force-fed or gentle pressure).

The length of this process also varies depending on whether the parent follows my feeding recommendations or whether they bend the rules. For example, offering baby a bottle-feed more often than recommended, or feeding baby while sleeping during the day. At best, bending the rules will prolong the process for who knows how long. At worst, it will prevent the process from working. (Chapter 14 describes reasons for lack of progress).

Keep track of baby's progress

Throughout the **adjustment period** – the time it takes to regain baby's trust and change her feelings about feeding from avoidance to delight – I encourage you to watch for certain markers to determine if things are on track. To identify these markers, I recommend the following strategies:

1. Record baby's fluid intake and output.

2. Rate her feeding behavior.

3. Compare baby's progress against 'What to expect'.

Let's look at each strategy in detail.

Record baby's fluid intake and output

You've probably already been keeping tack of how much your baby drinks and possibly how often she pees and poops. Continue this throughout the adjustment period.

You may find the table below helpful. But any way you choose to record what baby takes in and puts out will work. You might have an app on your phone.

Table 13.1: Fluids, wet diapers and behavior chart

Day:	Daily milk volume: Daily water volume:			Number of wet diapers: Bowel motions:				
Time	1st offer amount	Rating	2nd offer amount	Rating	Total amount	Pee	Poop

Milk

Your baby's milk intake will be one way you can assess her progress. Recording times and volumes will enable you to view her feeding pattern and consider how it compares from day to day.

Aim for your baby to receive a minimum of 10 ounces (300 ml) of **fluids** in a 24-hour period, providing sleep-feeds at night if necessary. Ideally, this will be all milk if baby is on regular strength breast milk or formula (20 kcal per ounce or 67 kcal per 100 ml), but a little less milk is fine if she's given high-energy feeds and has some water which takes her total fluids to around 10 ounces. Most babies don't drop this low, but a small percentage can.

While you can expect a significant drop in baby's milk intake when you first change your feeding practices, it shouldn't remain as low for more than a couple of days. Milk intake will **gradually** increase over the adjustment period, but not in a perfect linear pattern. There will be ups and downs, but overall improvement.

Water

Keep track of how much water baby drinks. If your baby's milk intake falls below 10 ounces in a 24-hour period, include her water intake in the fluid estimation.

Urine

Keep a close check on how often your baby pees. Even a small pee (as evidenced by a lightly damp diaper) counts as a pee, check and change her diaper regularly, even if her diapers are only slightly damp.

How often your baby pees will provide some indication of her hydration level. Five or more wet diapers in a 24-hour period means she's adequately hydrated at present. Three to four wet diapers in 24 hours means she's mildly dehydrated. This won't harm a physically healthy baby in the short-term. Babies often become mildly dehydrated when they're unwell, and for a much longer period than might occur during the adjustment period.

I find around 75 percent of babies going through this process don't drop lower than four wet diapers. Twenty percent might have three wet diapers for a day, and five percent drop to three wet diapers for two days. If the number of times your baby pees was to drop to three wet diapers in 24-hours, aim to increase the fluids she receives, but without pressure. This might involve water or milk via a syringe, spoon or cup, one or two sleep-feeds at night, or as a last resort a sleep-feed in the day.

Bowel motions

Baby will likely drink less milk in the early stages as a result of pressure being removed and stopping daytime sleep-feeds and/or spoon or syringe feeding of milk. And so she's probably not going to poop as often as usual. It's uncommon for a baby to become constipated during this process, but it can happen in a small percentage of babies. If your baby is prone to constipation, you need to watch out for this. If you suspect she's constipated provide the usual treatment or ask her doctor to recommend treatment.

Rating baby's feeding behavior

Your baby's progress is not based solely on how much milk she drinks. The main purpose of responding to her cues of interest and disinterest in feeding is to encourage her to enjoy feeding. Once this happens, she will consume enough milk to support healthy growth. So signs that show she's starting to relax and enjoy feeding also indicate positive progress.

Refer to Table 13.2 and rate your baby's feeding behavior at each feed. Compare behavioral ratings from day to day to monitor her progress. **Note:** Ratings are based on **behavior only** and not the amount of milk taken.

Table 13.2: Feeding behavior ratings

5	Feeds in a relaxed manner ends the feed in a passive way
4	Minor fussiness or distractibility while feeding ends the feed in a passive way
3	Appears restlessness throughout the feed ends the feed in a tense manner
2	Displays conflicted feeding behavior (see Chapter 1 for description); cries during the feed ends the feed abruptly in a distressed manner
1	Screaming as soon as she realizes she's going to be offered a feed (as opposed to crying due to hunger) or when shown the bottle she rejects in distressed manner (as opposed to passive rejection because she's not hungry)

Now let's look at what you might expect in regards to your baby's milk intake and behavior ratings throughout the adjustment period.

What to expect

When I explain to parents what to expect, I like to describe how a strongly resistant baby might behave. That way, parents are not unduly alarmed if this is the case for their baby. However, I find most babies do better than I describe. I encourage you to expect your baby to be strongly resistant. If she is, you're prepared. If she's not, then you can be pleasantly surprised when she does better than you're expecting.

Below I describe typical behavior at different stages during the adjustment period. Please bear in mind that not all babies will behave **exactly** as described.

Day 1

Feeding behavior ratings (as per Table 13.2) are typically 1 and 2. Baby will be apprehensive or fearful of feeding at this point. Past experiences have taught her that she's going to be pressured, and so as soon as she recognizes she's about to be fed she becomes tense or upset in anticipation.

If strongly averse to feeding, she will reluctantly accept a feed only when she's ravenous. It could take **many** hours for her to reach that point. She might reject a number of feeds in a row, possibly only willingly accepting your offer of a feed around mid to late afternoon.

Even when she finally accepts the bottle, she's going to be very tense and hyper vigilant in expectation of being pressured. She eats quickly, taking only enough to ease the discomfort caused by hunger pangs before abruptly stopping, at which point she becomes upset, because she's expecting pressure. If anything disturbs her, she might stop sucking sooner. She can be easily put off eating by any sudden movement of the person feeding her, or unexpected noise.

Her total daily milk intake will be at the lowest point of this process. (Note: A small percentage of babies' lowest point is on Day 2 or 3.)

Between feeds, she will probably to be irritable and find it hard to go to sleep and stay asleep because of hunger. Yet despite feeling hungry, she's likely to reject multiple offers to feed her.

Upon seeing your precious baby rejecting feeds or taking so little despite being hungry, your anxiety levels will go through the roof. The urge to resort to your previous feeding methods, such as sleep-feeding, spoon or syringe feeding or pressuring her to feed will be strong.

Day 2

Behavioral ratings fluctuate between 1 and 3. Seventy-five percent of babies show **subtle signs** of improvement on Day 2. Your baby might reject morning feeds, but accepts feeds sooner in the day and take a little more over the course of the day compared to Day 1.

Note: In general, morning feeds improve last during this process.

Twenty-five percent of babies continue to display strongly oppositional feeding behavior on Day 2. In this group, there might **not** be visible signs of improvement, and baby's total daily intake could be similar or possibly lower compared to Day 1.

Either way baby goes, she's likely to be cranky between feeds and may have trouble sleeping.

Your anxiety levels will remain at a very high level as you fight the urge to return to old habits to make sure she eats.

Day 3

Ratings are mostly 2 and 3. The memory of being pressured is beginning to fade, and your baby is slowly starting to let down her guard. But she's still uneasy when offered feeds.

She's no longer screaming when placed into a feeding position or at the sight of a bottle, but could still be tense and upset. She's more willing to take the bottle when offered, but not every time it's offered. She might reject the first feed or two of the day, but cautiously accept offers to feed at other times.

You're going to feel confused when reading her feeding cues. She acts like she's conflicted between wanting and not wanting to feed. She takes a little milk and pushes the nipple out with her tongue or hands, or turns her head or arches back to break away. No sooner is the nipple out of her mouth and she wants it back again. If you were to return the bottle, she might take a few sips and spits it out again. (See Chapter 11 'What if baby looks like she wants it again after rejecting?' for recommendations on how to respond to conflicted feeding behavior.)

The amount of milk baby takes will vary considerably from feed to feed. She feeds better in the afternoon and evening compared to morning feeds. Her total daily milk intake will be a little higher than Day 1.

Don't panic if your baby's intake is **not** higher than Day 1. A small percentage of babies do better than expected on Day 1, and in these cases intake could be slightly lower on Day 3. If this happens, look for signs of improvement in regards to her feeding behavior to determine if things are on track.

You're now witnessing signs of improvement and so you're feeling a little more hopeful about this process working. But anticipatory anxiety, where you feel anxious when thinking about feeding your baby, remains high.

Decide whether to proceed

Day 3 is the time I would expect **all babies** to demonstrate that things are beginning to turn around. Some babies, but not all, may have already done so on Day 2. On Day 3 you need to decide whether to continue or stop.

- If there are **signs of improvement on Day 3**, proceed with the feeding recommendations, and continue to compare against my description of typical behavior during this process to confirm that baby's progress remains on track.
- If there are **no signs of improvement on Day 3**, it's usually because baby is still being pressured to feed, but there can be other reasons. See Chapter 14 for potential reasons for lack of progress.

Days 4–7

Ratings tend to be mostly 3, with some 2s and 4s. Baby has now had many days of not being pressured to feed, but she's not over her aversion yet.

She's now willingly accepting a feed **when hungry**. She might get upset if she's offered a feed before she's ready to eat. She might continue to display conflicted feeding behavior at times, but this is decreasing.

Progress occurs in a two steps forward, one back, two forward, and one back pattern. 'Step-back' days can occur at any time. Baby is a little more content between feeds and sleeping may have improved. If you're not seeing an overall pattern of improvement over time, read Chapter 14.

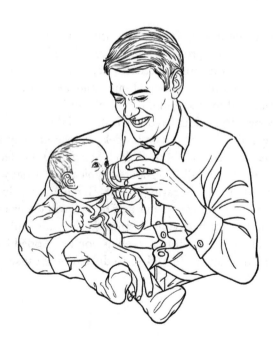

'Step-back' days

A step-back day means today baby is not feeding as well as she did yesterday. When these days occur – and they will – you'll probably feel alarmed. You will worry 'Is she regressing?' 'Am I doing something wrong?' 'Is this process not working?' 'Could there be an unidentified physical cause?' While baby's regression could be due to any one of these reasons, usually it's not. Step-back days typically occur due to tiredness.

When a baby is both tired and hungry, tiredness tends to win. So baby fusses more and feeds poorly. In the case of a step-back day due to tiredness, things are usually back on track the following day. Less often, baby might have two step-back days in a row.

Step-back days can also occur if baby becomes upset for any reason, such as illness, teething, or vaccinations. If these reasons are responsible, it can take longer for things to step forward again.

Days 8–14

Baby's feeding continues to improve. As the memory of being pressured fades she is becoming progressively more relaxed while feeding, but her receptiveness to feeding fluctuates depending on her mood, level of hunger and tiredness. Milk volumes and behavioral ratings also fluctuate from feed to feed and day to day, but in general both volume and receptiveness to feeding head in the desired direction.

At some point in the second week, baby willingly takes good volumes **over the course of the day**. She could be feeding more frequently than is generally considered typical for a baby of her age. The number of 4 and 5 ratings gradually increases in frequency. Progress can be slow and some ups and downs will occur in relation to her intake and feeding behavior. 'Step-back' days can still occur.

If your baby is not feeding as well as you had hoped by the end of two weeks, read Chapters 14 and 15 to discover the cause.

Undoubtedly, you have had your hopes raised in the past, so you'll be cautiously optimistic as you see the situation improving. It may take **many** weeks for you to feel confident that your baby is not going to suddenly revert to her previous aversive feeding behavior, before your anxiety levels drop.

Signs that baby is no longer averse

Your baby's milk intake and feeding behavior will help you determine when she's no longer averse to bottle-feeding.

Milk intake

Once over her aversion, your baby will willingly drink good volumes – sufficient for healthy growth – over the course of the day. This won't necessarily be the amount you think or have been told she needs. Health professionals sometimes overestimate a baby's milk needs. You might need to adjust your expectations. (See Chapter 6.)

While her total milk intake over a 24-hour period is good, her feeding pattern might not be what you expect for a baby of her age. Chapter 15 explains why this might occur and how to improve her feeding pattern.

Feeding behavior

Using Table 13.2 to rate her feeding behavior, she has behavioral ratings of mostly 4 and 5. Some fussiness and distractibility while feeding (rating 4) is normal infant behavior. As it's not always possible to prevent the clash of hunger and tiredness, she might occasionally feed in a way that warrants a rating of 3.

If she's not getting enough sleep at this stage, consider whether she needs sleep training to change negative sleep associations to positive ones.

If you have temporarily ceased solids, start to offer them again. (See Chapter 15 for recommendations on recommencing solids.)

Next we look at the reasons why this process might not be working as well as has been described.

14
It's not working!

> Everything you say about feeding Campbell while awake and letting him decide how much he eats makes sense. Yesterday I tried to follow your feeding rules, but I felt so stressed when he wouldn't eat. By the afternoon he was crying so hard because he was hungry. I knew he would eat in his sleep, so I fed him as he napped. The same thing happened today. I'm desperate to fix his feeding aversion but I don't think I can do this.
> – Brooke

In order to resolve a baby's behavioral feeding aversion, parents must first change the way they manage their baby's feeds. Without doing so they may continue to reinforce baby's avoidant feeding behavior. Brooke understood why Campbell's milk intake was expected to drop in the early days of following my feeding recommendations, and why he might choose to go hungry rather than eat while awake. But emotionally, she couldn't bear the increased anxiety this caused. By Day 2, she reverted to her previous custom of feeding Campbell as he slept during the day and night. Consequently, he continued to reject bottle-feeds while awake. This was not a case of my feeding recommendations not working; Brooke just felt she couldn't follow the rules.

While my **Five Steps to Success** are highly effective in resolving infant bottle-feeding aversions, not all babies get over their aversion.

The reasons for lack of improvement fit within the following categories:

- Breaking the rules
- Not following my recommendations and
- Physical or sensory reasons.

I recommend you read this chapter **before** making any changes to the way you currently manage your baby's feeds. Prior warning of the reasons others have stumbled could help improve your chances of successfully resolving your baby's feeding aversion.

If while following my feeding rules and recommendations, your baby's feeding doesn't progress as described in Chapter 13, return and reread this chapter.

Breaking the rules

My **Five Steps to Success** include four feeding **rules** and a number of **recommendations** designed to guide parents towards changing their infant feeding practices. By following these you can avoid accidently reinforcing baby's aversive feeding behavior, motivate baby to want to eat, and promote baby's enjoyment of bottle-feeding.

Golden feeding rules

1. No pressure to feed.
2. No sleep-feeding.
3. Bottle-feeds only.
4. Follow baby's lead.

These four feeding rules are **key strategies** to supporting a baby to change his feelings and desire to bottle-feed. The goal of these strategies is to guide him from wanting to avoid bottle-feeding and eating very little to enjoying feeding and eating enough for healthy growth. With a **few exceptions** the rules must be followed.

A baby's aversion does not suddenly resolve because parents change their feeding management. Milk intake is expected to drop in the early days of following my feeding recommendations.

In some cases, it will be a significant drop. Extreme anxiety experienced by parents when they witness this drop is usually the reason parents break these rules.

Breaking the 'no-pressure' rule

If pressure is the cause of your baby's feeding aversion, pressure will reinforce his aversion. Pressuring a baby to feed reminds him that feeding is an unpleasant or stressful experience and so it will strengthen his determination to avoid feeding.

There are **no exceptions** to the 'no pressure' rule. Pressuring your baby even once has the potential to cause a complete relapse, which would then mean starting from Day 1 over again.

Remember, there are various forms of 'pressure'. (See Chapter 3 for examples.) If your baby is not showing signs of progress by Day 3, confirm that you're not unintentionally pressuring him to accept feeds or continue eating.

If extreme anxiety prevents you from **consistently** following my 'no-pressure' feeding rule, consider allowing another of baby's caregivers to manage all his feeds until he's over his feeding aversion, then return to feeding him. I also recommend that you consider speaking with your healthcare professional about ways to manage your anxiety.

Breaking the 'no sleep-feeding' rule

When challenged by the reality of caring for a crying, hungry baby who fiercely opposes feeding, some parents resort to feeding their baby during sleep.

While I completely understand why a desperate parent would prefer to feed their baby during sleep than battle with him while awake, sleep-feeding provides only a temporary solution of making baby (and thus the parent) feel better at that moment. It doesn't solve the problem that's causing him to not want to eat while awake.

Once you start to follow my feeding plan, if you continue to provide sleep-feeds during the day your baby will probably continue to reject feeds while awake. This is because he might not get the chance to get hungry enough to override his opposition to feeding while awake. And there will be fewer opportunities for him to learn that he's now in control of how much he eats and that no one is going to pressure him. **Continued sleep-feeding will delay or prevent him from getting over his bottle-feeding aversion.**

Diagram 14.1: Sleep-feeding cycle

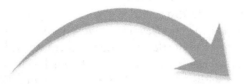

Parent feeds baby during sleep because he objects to feeding while awake.

Baby's hunger is satisfied during sleep-feeds enabling him to avoid feeding while awake.

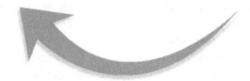

As you follow my 'no sleep-feeding' rule, at times you'll see your baby in a tired and hungry state. It's going to be difficult to resist an almost overwhelming urge to feed him as he's falling asleep or as he sleeps because you know his little body needs food and rest. But I encourage you to resist the temptation. To provide more incentive to stay on course, I list the disadvantages of sleep-feeding below, many of which you will already know:

1. It indirectly reinforces a baby's avoidance of feeding while awake.
2. It's extremely restrictive on family life.
3. It's not sustainable over the long term.
4. It can cause sleep deprivation if baby's sleep is disturbed as a result of trying to feed him.
5. It could disrupt baby's natural body rhythms if he feeds more often at night than he needs according to his stage of development.
6. It's associated with an increased risk of choking.
7. It's linked to tooth decay.

As you can see, there are a lot of good reasons to stop.

The advantage of sleep-feeding – that is, not battling with your baby to get him to feed – will no longer apply if you follow my feeding rules. There will be no feeding battles if you allow your baby to decide if he will eat or not. If he chooses not to, you need to respect his right to refuse and remove the bottle. Provided you consistently respond in harmony with his wishes (as demonstrated by his behavioral cues), his willingness to feed while awake will increase over time. The few days of upset due to hunger in the early stages of resolving his aversion to bottle-feeding will pass.

If you can't resist the temptation to feed your baby in a drowsy state or as he sleeps during the day, it may mean he doesn't get over his feeding aversion. You might find the 'Band-Aid' solutions described in Chapter 4 help to maintain his growth until he no longer requires bottle-feeding. But take care to avoid pressuring him to eat solid foods because this might cause him to become averse to eating solids as well.

Apart from the exception of providing sleep-feeds at night to ensure your baby receives the minimum daily milk intake of 10 ounces (300 ml), the 'no sleep-feeding' rule should ideally be adhered to. Some parents like to continue to provide their baby with one sleep-feed (sometimes called a dream feed) at night. One sleep-feed at night doesn't usually prevent a baby from getting over his aversion provided all other feeds are offered while awake.

Breaking the 'bottle-only' rule

If your baby rejects bottle-feeds or doesn't drink as much as you're hoping he will, it's going to be tempting to try to get him to take milk in another way, such as a sippy cup, spoon or syringe, or give him solids. However, I suggest you avoid doing so. Such measures will provide temporary relief from a hungry tummy, but they will do nothing to resolve his aversion to bottle-feeding. By satisfying his hunger using these means, you will remove his primary motivation to accept milk from a bottle, and in doing so delay or prevent him from getting over his aversion to bottle-feeding.

Feeding a baby in these ways is usually not sustainable over the long-term. Babies in general cannot handle drinking from a sippy cup before eight months of age and even then, few babies will drink volumes large enough for it to be the primary vessel for milk feeds. Giving milk from a spoon or syringe will involve a long and tedious process that will significantly hamper family life. And solids are a poor substitute for milk for a baby. Resolving your baby's aversion to bottle-feeding is the best solution.

Exceptions to the 'bottle-only' rule apply at night only. These ensure baby's basic needs are met. (See Chapter 10.)

Breaking the 'follow baby's lead' rule

Breaking the 'no pressure' rule means the 'follow baby's lead' rule is also broken because if you're pressuring your baby to feed you're not following his lead and not respecting his right to decide when and how much to eat. But a parent might **not** follow baby's lead in other ways, for example:

- Harassing baby with repeated offers when he's rejecting.
- Keeping a hungry, distressed baby waiting too long to offer a feed by trying to stick to scheduled feeding times.
- Waking baby to feed because it's 'time'.

I appreciate that the 'follow baby's lead' rule can be challenging because a baby might not give clear signals in the early stages of resolving his feeding aversion, a time he will still be apprehensive about feeding.

Don't try to stick with a time-based feeding schedule throughout this process. While my recommendation is to offer feeds three hourly or sooner if baby shows hunger cues, if baby happened to be napping at that time, leave him sleeping. Sleep is as important to a baby's health as food.

If you have ruled out other reasons for your baby's lack of progress described in this chapter, video yourself feeding baby and objectively assess your response to his feeding cues. Determine if you're responding in harmony with his cues or according to your feelings of anxiety.

Ask your partner, a family member or friend to provide some honest feedback; does he/she think you're offering too often or persisting too long to try to 'encourage' your baby to accept the bottle or continue eating?

Exceptions to 'follow baby's lead' rule

In some circumstances you may need to take the lead or respond in a way that doesn't appear to harmonize with baby's wishes. For example: You may need to ...

- Wake him during the night to offer milk or provide a feed during sleep to ensure he reaches the minimum daily amount.
- Stick to the 'two offers per feed' recommendation even if directly after rejecting your baby continues to display signs of hunger. This is so you don't harass him by repeated offers when he's showing you he's not willing to eat.
- Remove the bottle if he shows conflicted feeding behavior – even though he appears to want it again immediately after rejecting – to avoid reinforcing this behavior. (Explained further in the next section.)
- Prevent him from falling asleep while feeding – even though he appears to desperately want to fall asleep while sucking on a bottle, as occurs in the case of feeding-sleep association – to resolve his bottle-feeding aversion. (Also explained further in the next section.)

Not following feeding recommendations

Throughout the chapters in Part C, I have made a number of recommendations, which I'll list here, plus a few extra tips.

Feeding recommendations summary
- Ensure there are no sucking, positioning or airflow problems before starting this process. (See Chapter 2.)
- Don't try to put the bottle into baby's mouth without his permission.
- Quickly remove the bottle away from baby's line of sight at the first sign of rejection.

- Don't linger with the bottle in front of baby's face if he's rejecting. This can torment a baby who is apprehensive or fearful of feeding.
- Offer only twice per feed. If your baby consistently rejects the second offer, then offer only once.
- Avoid tactics that involve coercion, cajoling, or trickery to make baby eat or continue eating when he wants to stop. (See Chapter 3 for examples.)
- Don't add bitter tasting medication to baby's bottle.
- Discourage a feeding-sleep association, where baby relies on feeding as a way to fall asleep.
- Discourage conflicted feeding behavior by removing the bottle when baby turns away. Go for a break or end the feed.
- Avoid situations that might stress baby.
- Feed baby in a quiet environment while he displays signs of tension while feeding.
- Limit the number of people feeding baby, ideally to one person.
- Plan to be home for the first three days to support baby's sleep, as this will be the time he's likely to feel hunger and yet rejects feeds and therefore find it difficult to sleep.
- Aim for all feeds to be offered at home during the adjustment period.
- Try to maintain a regular wake-up time for baby in the mornings to help stabilize his internal body clock.

These are not rules that must be adhered to, but rather suggested ways to make feeding easier or more acceptable for a baby throughout the adjustment period.

You might feel that these recommendations are not necessary or might not fit well within your family's circumstances, for example others might need to feed your baby while you're working.

You may find you can deviate from these recommendations and still witness an improvement in your baby's aversive feeding behavior. However, if things are not going well, I encourage you to reconsider any recommendation that you're not currently following.

While all of these recommendations can help improve the chances of a baby getting over his feeding aversion, there are two recommendations which if not followed are more likely to inhibit progress. These are: discourage conflicted feeding behavior and a feeding-sleep association. The responses I recommend in these circumstances are exceptions to the 'follow baby's lead' rule. I explain the reasons below.

Discourage conflicted feeding behavior

> He cried when I took the bottle away. It feels so mean to do this when he wants it. He drinks more if I keep giving it back to him. – Emma

Conflicted feeding behavior is when baby takes a few mouthfuls, breaks away **in a tense manner**, comes back, wants the bottle, takes a few mouthfuls, breaks away, comes back, wants the bottle and so on. My recommendation is to remove the bottle when baby turns away, and go for a break or end the feed so as to not reinforce this behavior. (See 'What if baby looks like she wants it again after rejecting' in Chapter 11 for further explanation.)

Most parents find this difficult to do. And understandably so. It doesn't feel right to remove the bottle when baby indicates he wants it back again. Hence some parents ignore my recommendation to remove the bottle and instead continue to reoffer the bottle each time baby returns after breaking away. But then find their baby continues to feed in an unsettled conflicted manner well beyond the time estimated for his feeding aversion to be resolved.

While it **might** be okay to keep returning the bottle, it **might not**. If your baby's conflicted feeding behavior has **not** been reinforced, it should fade during the early days and disappear by around Day 5, if not before. If your baby continues to display strongly conflicted behavior on Day 6 and beyond, this may indicate that this disjointed tense feeding behavior has been reinforced.

If you have accidentally reinforced your baby's conflicted feeding behavior and now decide to correct this situation by following my recommendation to remove the bottle when he first turns away, expect this to cause a drop in his milk intake in the short-term. It may also mean it takes longer than the estimated two-week period for him to get over his aversion if you have not being doing so from Day 1.

Discourage a feeding-sleep association

Another reason why parents might not witness signs of improvement is if they don't follow my recommendation to discourage their baby's feeding-sleep association. (Sleep associations are explained in Chapter 12.) The reason some parents don't follow these recommendations is because their baby doesn't know how to fall asleep without feeding to sleep. And they don't want to upset baby by preventing him from doing so.

When a baby learns to rely on feeding **as a way to fall asleep** this means he will appear hungry and want to suck on a bottle whenever he's tired. However, if he's allowed to fall asleep while sucking on a bottle, then it's not going to be possible to follow the 'no sleep-feeding' rule. As already explained, if he feeds in a drowsy or sleepy state this can delay or prevent him from getting over his feeding aversion. So nothing may change.

To discourage a feeding-sleep association involves more than following the 'no sleep-feeding' rule. Preventing your baby from falling asleep while bottle-feeding aims to change his dependence on feeding as a way to fall asleep. He can learn to fall asleep in a new way with your guidance and support. (See Chapter 12 for more.)

Physical and sensory reasons

Sometimes parents follow **all** my feeding rules and recommendations and their baby doesn't progress as expected. Some reasons for this include:

- Physical problems.
- Highly sensitive baby.
- Major or minor sucking problems (described in Chapter 2).
- Sensory processing disorder.

Physical problems

Any physical problem – whether illness, a medical condition or disorder – that has the potential to cause loss of appetite, discomfort or pain, could impede a baby's progress. Chapter 4 describes medical reasons for babies to become averse to feeding, such as acid reflux, milk allergy or intolerance. The potential of these problems needs to be assessed, and if necessary treated, **before** using my **Five Steps to Success.**

During the two weeks or so that it takes for a baby to get over his feeding aversion following my feeding rules and recommendations, he could experience an illness or physical problem that inhibits his progress or causes a minor or major setback. For example, teething, constipation, infective illness such as a respiratory, gastro-intestinal or urinary tract infection, an adverse reaction to vaccinations or due to the side effects of medications.

If you suspect your baby is troubled by teething discomfort or constipation, these problems can generally be treated quickly with only a minor setback and you can continue to follow my feeding rules and recommendations.

However, if you're worried about illness or a more serious physical problem, ask a doctor to examine your baby. If your baby is unwell or has a problem that's likely to cause pain or loss of appetite return to your previous feeding practices – with the **exception** of upsetting your baby by trying to pressure him to feed – and wait until the problem is treated or resolved before trying again.

Highly sensitive baby

Around five percent of babies who are averse to feeding are highly sensitive to pressure. These babies don't respond well to being offered more than once per feed, or to the parent lingering too long with the bottle in baby's sight, or to being held in a feeding position after he rejects the bottle.

My theory is that being offered more than once could be perceived by a sensitive baby as pressure, even though the parent is merely offering a second time. And that by lingering with the bottle within baby's line of sight or maintaining him in a feeding position after he rejects it, may cause him to feel threatened that he will be made to feed using pressure tactics – like he was in the past – even though the parent has no intention of doing so.

To resolve a highly sensitive baby's feeding aversion, the parent needs to offer once only at each feed. And quickly remove the bottle out of baby's sight and remove him from a feeding position at the slightest hint of rejection.

Sensory processing disorder

A sensory processing disorder is **one of the least likely** causes of feeding aversion. But it is a cause. A sensory processing disorder means the stimulus causing baby's aversive feeding behavior could be the feel, taste or sensations associated with feeding. (See Chapter 1 for more.) If this is the case, baby's aversive feeding behavior may continue to be reinforced despite parents following my feeding rules and recommendations.

Based on feeding behavior alone, it's virtually impossible for a health professional to tell the difference between infant distress which occurs in response to a pressure-induced feeding aversion and distress due to a sensory processing problem. Therefore, it's imperative to eliminate **the most likely** cause – pressure – before assuming baby's aversive behavior occurs as a result of **the least likely cause** – a sensory processing disorder.

Remember, it can take weeks for a baby to recover from a pressure-related feeding aversion after **all** pressure is removed, subtle and obvious. Plus, as you have already learned from reading this book, the successful resolution of a baby's feeding aversion usually requires much more than simplistically advising parents to remove pressure.

Where to find support

If you're confident you have followed my Five Steps to Success – all rules and recommendations – and have not witnessed any indication of improvement by Day 3, consult with baby's doctor to rule out physical causes and if further assessment of sensory processing disorder is needed.

If your baby is well, consider an assessment and ongoing support throughout this process from a professional experienced in baby feeding aversions through my Baby Care Advice website: www.babycareadvice.com.

In the next chapter we look at life after your baby's feeding aversion is resolved.

15
Life after baby's aversion

> I am not sure whether Claire is over her aversion or not. She seems to like eating now. She's excited to see the bottle, but she only takes 2 to 3 ounces (60-90 ml) before she calmly pushes the nipple out like she's saying 'I am done now.' Then she wants to feed again an hour or two later. So she's having about 10 feeds a day. Is that normal? I thought she would be eating bigger amounts by now? – Kylie

I ask Kylie how much milk Claire is drinking in total each day. It's a good amount for a baby of her age and size. Kylie rates Claire's feeding behavior as mostly 5 out of 5. It appears like she's over her feeding aversion, which means Kylie can look beyond this issue for other ways to improve Claire's frequent feeding pattern.

Parents are ecstatic once they see their baby enjoying bottle-feeding. A HUGE weight has been lifted from their shoulders. The constant stress of trying to get their baby to eat is gone and they feel they can finally enjoy their baby. But it's not sunshine and roses for every family. Some parents have further work ahead to improve their baby's feeding patterns, or fix a sleeping problem, or resolve baby's aversion to eating solid foods.

Other parents might worry that their baby is not eating enough or not gaining as much weight as they expect. Usually the problem lies with their expectations rather than it being a real issue. However, a baby could be over her aversion to bottle-feeding and not eat quite enough. Other reasons why a baby may not eat as much as she needs are described in this chapter.

If things are not as good as they could be after your baby's feeding aversion is resolved, there may be additional steps you can take to support her to feed better and achieve her growth potential.

Concerns

Some parents have questions or concerns after baby gets over her bottle-feeding aversion. These are the most common:

1. Baby is feeding better, but not great.

2. Baby only feeds well for one parent.

3. Baby is not drinking as much as expected.

4. Baby is not gaining as much weight as expected.

5. How do I prevent a relapse?

6. When and how do I recommence solids?

7. How do I resolve baby's aversion to eating solids?

If you have any of these questions or concerns, please read this entire chapter because often there's a connection between the causes. If you don't have any concerns, then I suggest you read it anyway! Who knows when such concerns could present? Prior knowledge could spare you and your baby from needless anguish.

Baby is feeding is better, but not great

An aversion is not the only reason for a baby to fuss while feeding. So resolving your baby's bottle-feeding aversion doesn't guarantee that she's going to feed like a champion. Or that her feeding pattern will be ideal for a baby of her age.

Like any problem, the solution needs to address the cause. The following problems can negatively impact on a baby's feeding patterns and contentment while feeding:

- sleeping problem
- snack feeding
- excessive night feeding.

Sleeping problem

A baby's sleeping patterns influence her feeding patterns. If your baby's sleep is often broken – she wakes too soon still tired and grumpy – because of an underlying sleeping problem, she may want to feed more frequently. If she's not getting enough sleep she could become cranky due to sleep deprivation. Sleep deprivation will lower her frustration tolerance while feeding. She might not be willing to eat when offered a feed because she's too tired, but at the same time find it difficult to fall asleep because she's still hungry.

Preventing the clash of hunger and tiredness, by resolving any underlying sleeping problem, is going to be far more effective than trying to get an overtired baby to eat and a hungry baby to fall asleep.

If your baby's sleeping issues are due to a sleep association problem, then the current situation may not get better unless you take steps to improve her sleep. (See Chapter 12 for recommendations.)

Snack-feeding

If your baby's **total daily intake** and feeding behavior are good (mostly 4 and 5 ratings according to Table 13.2 in Chapter 13) this means she's over her feeding aversion. If she is then feeding more often than you would expect for her age, she may have developed a pattern of snack-feeding (ie taking frequent small feeds). One reason could be an underlying sleeping problem causing broken sleep. Another is that snack-feeding can occur out of habit – yours or baby's.

Snacking can become a cyclical pattern. The more frequently you offer your baby a feed, the less she needs to take – the less she takes, the more often she wants to feed.

Diagram 15.1: Snack-feeding cycle

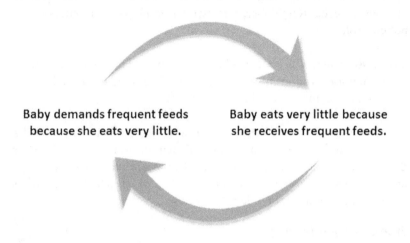

Baby demands frequent feeds
because she eats very little.

Baby eats very little because
she receives frequent feeds.

Snack feeding won't harm your baby, but it may mean she's feeding **more often** than she actually needs. If you're happy to continue, you don't need to do anything different. But don't expect her to drink larger amounts per feed. Infant feeding patterns, like infant behavior, are reinforced by the actions parents take. If you would like your baby to take larger volumes less often, then you may need to lead her towards this goal. Try the following steps:

Step 1: Check that you have realistic expectations about the number of feeds that are reasonable for a baby of her age.

Table 15.1: Average number of bottle-feeds for age

Age	24-hour period
Birth–1 month	6–8
1–3 months	6
3–6 months	5
6–9 months	4
9–12 months	3

Some babies will feed more or less often. More feeds might be necessary if your baby has catch-up growth to achieve. Use these figures as a general guide but don't try to make her stick to a set number of feeds. Remember, effective parenting is about support and not control.

Step 2: Resolve any sleeping problem baby might have. This may enable her to nap longer, and in doing so, naturally extend the time between feeds, resulting in larger volumes at each feed.

Step 3: Gradually stretch the time between her feeds to intervals that range between three to four hours, depending on her age. Start by delaying the time you offer her a feed by 15-minute increments and entertain her while she waits. But don't try to stretch the time if she becomes upset and is not able to be soothed.

Excessive night feeding

Excessive night feeding refers to a situation where a baby feeds more often than required at her stage of development. By night, I am referring to a 12-hour period, eg seven pm to seven am. **During** the night meaning the number of times baby wakes to be fed or is offered a sleep-feed **after** being settled for the night, and **not** counting the feed prior to bedtime.

Whether or not a baby feeds excessively **during the night** would depend on how often she wakes to feed or is fed while sleeping. Table 15.2 lists the average number of night feeds for age.

Table 15.2: Average number of night feeds for age

Age	Number of feeds DURING the night
Birth–3 months	2
3–6 months	1
6+ months	0

Of course individuals differ for various reasons. A feeding aversion can cause some babies to gain weight poorly. Your baby might need to feed more often if she has some catch-up growth to achieve once her aversion is resolved.

If your baby's total daily intake is good, and she's mostly enjoying feeding while awake, but she doesn't seem hungry or interested in feeding in the mornings, this could indicate that she's feeding more often than she needs during the night.

A pattern of excessive feeding at night can develop **prior to or while** resolving baby's feeding aversion. You might have previously resorted to sleep-feeding your baby multiple times during the night to try to increase her daily milk intake. Or prior to or during the process of resolving her feeding aversion, she might have woken to demand extra feeds at night because her milk intake during the day was low. After resolving her feeding aversion the pattern of feeding often at night might continue because the frequent night feeding pattern has caused her circadian rhythms (24-hour internal body clock) to become out of sync with a normal day-night feeding pattern.

Effects

Our circadian rhythms influence appetite through the release of hormones such as leptin, which suppresses appetite, and ghrelin, which stimulates appetite. The reason we don't eat at night is because our appetite is suppressed due to the effects of leptin. As babies mature they go for longer periods at night without eating because leptin is released for longer periods. From a developmental perspective, most babies' circadian rhythms have matured enough to enable them to go for around eight hours at night without eating by three months, and 10–12 hours by six months of age.

When a baby feeds more often at night than necessary according to her stage of development, this can cause a shift in hormone release. The period of reduced appetite that would ideally occur at night gets pushed into the morning. And as a result she then rejects or eats very little in the mornings, not appearing hungry until late morning or early afternoon, but eats well after that time.

A cyclical pattern can establish. The more she eats at night, the less she needs to eat the following day – the less she eats during the day, the more likely she will wake to demand feeds at night to make up for any short-fall.

Diagram 15.2: Dysrhythmic day-night feeding cycle

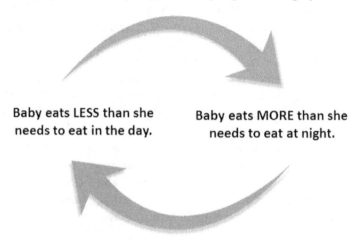

Baby eats LESS than she
needs to eat in the day.

Baby eats MORE than she
needs to eat at night.

This cycle won't necessarily change in the short term unless you encourage a shift in her day-night feeding pattern. The following steps might encourage her to eat more in the day and less often at night.

Step 1: If you have not already done so, cease sleep-feeding at night. Feeding a baby during sleep will encourage night feedings she might not need. Only offer her a feed at night if she wakes to demand it.

Step 2: Make sure your baby is not reliant on negative sleep associations (see Chapter 12), as these will increase the likelihood of her waking in the night. You might then assume she's waking due to hunger when in reality she's waking naturally between sleep cycles as we all do at times during the night, and she's then crying because she has learned to rely on your help or certain props to go to sleep. In particular, prevent her from falling asleep while bottle-feeding both during the day and night. While she's reliant on feeding as a way to fall asleep, she's likely to want to feed in the night to return to sleep.

Step 3: Gradually reduce the amount of milk you offer your baby at night and eliminate extra night feeds one at a time. Don't try to go below the average number of night feeds for age. As a result of eliminating extra night feeds, she'll start to get hungrier and eat more in the mornings. But don't expect a direct correlation between the amount reduced at night and amount increased the next day. It can take a few days for her circadian rhythms to adjust.

Baby only feeds well for one parent

When one parent provides all or most feeds to support baby through the process of resolving her feeding aversion, baby learns that this parent will provide an appropriate response to her feeding cues. As the parent regains her trust she starts to relax and enjoy feeding when this parent provides feeds. If she's not as willing to feed from her other parent or caregiver she may not yet have had sufficient opportunities to learn to trust that others will respond to her cues, and so she's apprehensive when others feed her.

If you find this to be the case, choose a time when the other parent or caregiver can provide **all feeds** over a number of consecutive days. Expect some resistance initially on baby's part. She might reject some feeds and her milk intake might drop in the short term. Basically, it means going through this process again with the other parent or another caregiver. However, she will turn around sooner, typically a couple of days, as she gains confidence that others will also respond according to her cues. That is provided you (or her main caregiver if that's not you) avoid the temptation to step in and take over when she resists feeds offered by others.

If you keep taking over because you know she's more willing to feed when you offer, it will probably take longer for her to feel confident that the other parent or caregiver is going to respond to her feeding cues. She might also learn that if she fusses or refuses to eat from others, you will feed her. Whether this is problematic or not depends on your family's circumstances.

Baby is not drinking as much as expected

Once your baby's feeding aversion is resolved, she might not drink as much as you're expecting. In this case I recommend the following steps:

Step 1: Check if baby shows signs of illness. If so, have her medically assessed.

Step 2: Check that she's over her feeding aversion. (See Chapter 13 for signs.)

Step 3: Check if she shows signs of being well fed.

- If **she's well fed**, check your expectations. Perhaps you're expecting her to drink more than she needs or her healthcare provider has overestimated her milk needs. Also consider if she could be going through a period of 'catch-down' growth, in which case she may not need the amount estimated using standard calculations based on age and weight. (See Chapter 7 for more on catch-down growth.)
- If **she doesn't appear to be well fed**, but she's physically well, rule out common reasons for underfeeding such as sleep deprivation, equipment problems and rigid feeding schedules. Also consider the possibility of other causes such as teething, change of routine, stress (eg, starting daycare or nursery, a new caregiver, vaccinations) and excitement (eg, visitors in the house, and traveling). If you're still concerned, have baby medically assessed.

Sometimes you can identify the reason why baby is not drinking as much as expected and remedy the situation, and sometimes you can't. In most instances, the cause will pass within a few days.

At times your baby's appetite may wane, perhaps due to the reasons mentioned or a plateau in growth (see Chapter 7), and she will take less milk than you expect. At other times she'll eat more than you expect. If you trust in her inborn ability to self-regulate her dietary intake, it will balance out. So please stay patient, follow her lead and see what happens regarding her weight gains and growth patterns over the next few weeks.

Whatever the cause, avoid pressuring her to feed, as this will likely reignite her feeding aversion and make the situation worse.

Baby is not gaining as much weight as expected

Don't forget that a baby is expected to lose a little weight during the process of resolving her feeding aversion. And she might not regain this for one to two weeks – provided her feeding aversion is resolved by that time.

Typically when a baby is **not** gaining as expected after resolving her feeding aversion the problem lies with expectations. It's normal for weight gains to fluctuate from week to week, and for a baby's weight to wander between percentile curves on an infant growth chart.

If after resolving your baby's feeding aversion she does **not gain** as much as you or her healthcare provider expects, **avoid making**

assumptions about the cause. Altering the way you manage her feeds or making changes to her diet without a complete understanding of the cause only serves to complicate the situation.

If your baby is not growing as expected, I recommend the following:

Step 1: Look for signs that show if your baby is well fed. (See Chapter 6.)

- **If she shows signs of being a well-fed baby,** there's probably nothing to worry about. In this case, see normal variations of growth in Chapter 7.
- **If she doesn't show signs of being well fed,** then she may not be over her feeding aversion or she may be underfeeding because of other reasons. (See Chapter 5.)

Step 2: If you're still concerned have her medically assessed.

Relapse prevention

Now that you have resolved your baby's feeding aversion, it doesn't mean you can go back to pressuring her to take more than she's willing to eat. You need to stick to your role when feeding her, that is, offer feeds either upon request or at intervals appropriate for her stage of development if she's a non-demanding baby, and respect her right to decide if she will accept your offer and how much she will eat. If you were to return to pressuring her, even in a gentle way, there's a high risk that she will relapse and once again become averse to bottle-feeding.

A complete relapse can occur after being pressured only once. And it could take a further two weeks or so to regain her trust and resolve the problem a second time. So trying to make her drink that extra ounce (30ml) left in the bottle is just not worth it.

Solids

You might have a number of questions about solids at this point. For example:

- When can I start baby back on solids?
- How can I prevent baby from becoming averse to eating solids?
- How do I resolve baby's aversion to eating solids?

When to recommence solids

Once your baby's bottle-feeding aversion is resolved it will be time to return to offering her solid foods, if she was eating solids previously. Otherwise wait until she's old enough to eat solids – usually between the ages of four and six months. Baby's healthcare provider will guide you.

To be sure that bottle-feeding doesn't get thrown out of kilter because of solids, I recommend you take things slowly to find the right balance. Initially offer her solids around 20–30 minutes **after** her bottle-feed. Start with one meal, watch for any impact on her milk intake, if there's no significant drop then offer twice the next day. Monitor the impact of two meals, then offer three, and so on.

Expect a drop in milk intake as a result of calories received from solids. How big this drop will be depends on the calorie content of the food and how much she eats. Once you feel confident that solids are not having an undesirable effect on her acceptance of bottle-feeds or a dramatic drop in milk intake, then decide whether to continue to offer solids after bottle-feeds or reverse the order. My recommendation is milk first until nine months of age and then decide which order works best for your baby to maintain a healthy balance between milk and solids.

Preventing and resolving an aversion to solids

Babies can become averse to eating solids for many of the same reasons that they become averse to bottle-feeding. The number 1 reason is because they're pressured to eat. Your baby has already demonstrated she doesn't take kindly to being pressured to feed from a bottle. So there's a good chance she could develop an aversion to solids if you were to try to make her eat against her will.

You have the same responsibilities when feeding your baby solid foods as you do when bottle-feeding. You're responsible for offering her nutritious foods at regular intervals appropriate for her stage of development. It's **not** your job to make sure she eats a specific amount.

Allow your baby to decide if she will accept what you offer and how much she will eat. Respond to her cues of interest or disinterest (described in Table 15.3) and make sure you don't apply pressure, or use cajoling, coercion, trickery or distractions to get her to accept the food you offer or eat more than she's willing to eat. Give her lots of opportunities to self-feed safe food (those that don't pose a choking risk) starting from around six months of age.

Table 15.3: Interest and disinterest in solids

Interest or receptiveness	Disinterest or rejection
<ul><li>Excited by sight of food.</li><li>Watches spoon approaching.</li><li>Leaning toward food.</li><li>Open mouth.</li><li>Accepting spoon/food into mouth.</li><li>Closing mouth around spoon/food.</li><li>Sucking or chewing food.</li><li>Swallowing food.</li><li>Self-feeding.</li></ul>	<ul><li>Refusing to get into high chair.</li><li>Getting upset when offered food.</li><li>Turning head or body away from food.</li><li>Arching back to distance self from food.</li><li>Clamped mouth.</li><li>Refusal to accept spoon/food into mouth.</li><li>Holding food in mouth without swallowing.</li><li>Spitting food out of mouth.</li></ul>

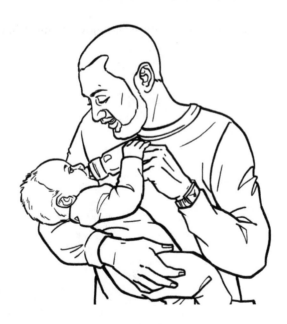

Congratulations

You have now resolved your baby's feeding aversion – a mammoth task. Well done! You have patiently and lovingly guided your baby from avoiding to enjoying feeding. It has undoubtedly been a tumultuous journey for you, your baby and family. There have been highs and lows. But you hung in there when the going got tough and your baby and family are now reaping the rewards and enjoying a more harmonious family life, free from the stress of trying to make your baby feed.

You might still worry about your baby's feeding at this stage. This is normal. It's because you have been under extreme stress for weeks or months. Even now that her aversion is over you're probably feeling a little anxious when feeding her, worried that she might not take the bottle or that you might unknowingly pressure her and cause a relapse. At times she might refuse or take only a little and this will heighten your fears of her aversion returning. The anxiety you feel will fade in time as you become more confident that she's not going to relapse.

You and your baby are now on the same page, each sticking to your individual responsibilities in the feeding partnership. Your baby is now enjoying eating as a result and growing well. Rest in that knowledge.

I wish you all the best for a future of enjoyable mealtimes with your child.

Rowena

References

[i] R Bryant-Waugh, L Markham, RE Kreipe, BT Walsh, 'Feeding and eating disorders in childhood', *International Journal of Eating Disorders*, March 2010, 43(2), pp 98–111.

[ii] RE Behrman, R Kliegman and HB Jenso HB (eds), *Nelson Textbook of Pediatrics*, 16th ed, WB Saunders, Philadelphia, 2000, pp 1125–26.

[iii] R Meyer, 'New guidelines for managing cow's milk allergy in infants', *Journal of Family Health*, 2008, 18(1), pp 27–30.

[iv] A Host and S Halken, 'Cow's milk allergy: Where have we come from and where are we going?', *Endocrine, Metabolic Immune Disorders – Drug Targets*, 2014 March 14(1), pp 2–8.

[v] Meyer, 'New guidelines for managing ...', pp 27–30.

[vi] A Host, 'Frequency of cow's milk allergy in childhood', *Annals of Allergy, Asthma and Immunology*, 2002, 89 (Suppl 1), pp 33–37.

[vii] GR Fleisher and S Ludwig, *Synopsis of Pediatric Emergency Medicine*, 4th ed, 2002, Lippincott Williams & Wilkins, Philadelphia, p 98.

[viii] Host and Halken, 'Cow's milk allergy...', pp 2–8.

[ix] Prilosec Side Effects Center, http://www.rxlist.com/prilosec-side-ef-fects-drug-center.htm (accessed 10 February 2017).

[x] N Van Herwaarden, JM Bos, B Veldman and C Kramers, 'Proton pump inhibitors: Not as safe as they seem', *Netherlands Tijdschrift voor Geneeskunde*, 2016, 160(0), D487.

[xi] E Satter, 'Division of Responsibility in Feeding', Ellyn Satter Institute, http://ellynsatterinstitute.org/dor/divisionofresponsibilityinfeeding.php (accessed 10 February 2017).

[12] National Health and Medical Research Council, *Infant Feeding Guidelines*, 2013, http://www.nhmrc.gov.au/_files_nhmrc/publications/attachments/n56_infant_feeding_guidelines.pdf (accessed 10 February 2017), p 79.

[13] Merck Manual, *Nutrition in Infants*, https://www.merckmanuals.com/professional/pediatrics/care-of-newborns-and-infants/nutrition-in-infants#v1076566 (accessed 10 February 2017).

[14] Breastfeeding Association, *Guide to Bottle Feeding*, https://www.breastfeeding.asn.au/system/files/UKHealthGuideBottlefeeding.pdf (accessed 13 September 2016).

[15] The British Dietetic Association (BDA), Food Fact Sheet: Complementary foods (weaning), May 2016. https://www.bda.uk.com/foodfacts/WeaningYourChild.pdf (accessed 23 February 2017).

[16] York Community Health Service, Canada, *Healthy Beginnings: Infant formula*, p 8, https://www.york.ca/wps/wcm/connect/yorkpublic/2a39389e-2d70-4f30-8b49-a6e3bab4859a/Feeding_Your_Baby_Infant_Formula.pdf?MOD=AJPERES (accessed 13 September 2016).

[17] https://www.cdc.gov/mmwr/preview/mmwrhtml/rr5909a1.htm (accessed 13 September 2016).

Index

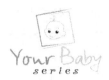

Your Baby
series

CPSIA information can be obtained
at www.ICGtesting.com
Printed in the USA
LVHW020124120721
692048LV00005B/29